The Nurse

in Radiology

The complete Guide

ALEXANDRE CAREWELL

Table of contents

« Radiology: where we take internal selfies to see if everything's in place inside ! »

Introduction:

Foreword: Why this book?

Radiology, that vast expanse of invisible waves, mysterious images and innovative techniques, is much more than just a series of medical examinations. It is the window through which contemporary medicine looks to understand, diagnose and, ultimately, heal. At the heart of this constantly evolving field are the radiology nurses, the real pillars of this often little-known medical world.

This book was born of a passion and a burning desire to shed light on the unique, but oh-so-rewarding, journey of these professionals. At a time when technology is evolving at breakneck speed and new techniques and approaches are emerging every day, it is crucial to have a reliable guide that is rooted in the day-to-day reality of these nurses.

So why this particular book? Firstly, because it aims to fill a gap. Although the medical literature is full of books on various specialities, few of them really dwell on the specific role and challenges of radiology nurses. This book is an ode to their dedication, a testament to their expertise, and above all, a tool for all those who wish to follow in their footsteps.

What's more, it's not just a book of theory. It is based on real stories, real experiences, hardships overcome and victories celebrated. It offers a candid look at what it means to be a radiology nurse, from the first hesitant steps of a novice to the complex challenges faced by veterans of the field.

Finally, throughout its pages, this book aims to encourage, inspire and guide. Whether you're a student, a novice or a seasoned professional, it's designed with you in mind. To remind you why you chose this path, to show you how much you can achieve, and to ensure that, whatever the challenges ahead, you are never alone.

Happy reading, and welcome to the fascinating world of radiology through the eyes of those who live it every day.

Radiology: An invisible world revealed

Behind the walls of hospitals, behind the scenes in medicine, lies a dimension where the invisible becomes palpable, where the unknown is revealed and where magic meets science. This is the realm of radiology, a discipline that has transformed the art of diagnosis and treatment, allowing us to travel inside the human body without the need for the slightest incision.

Imagine a world where we can see a child's heartbeat before it is even born, detect a tumour in its early stages of development or visualise the intricacies of the blood vessels that run through our brains. It's a world that could easily belong to a fantasy tale, but it's actually the everyday life of radiology professionals.

Although radiology was once regarded as a simple auxiliary branch of medicine, over the decades it has become one of its cornerstones. Through constant technological advances, it has become not only a diagnostic tool, but also a therapeutic one, changing the lives of millions of people around the world.

But what makes radiology so special, so unique? Perhaps it's its ability to reveal the invisible, to make the intangible

tangible. While our natural senses have their limits, radiology transcends them, offering us an almost superhuman vision of our own bodies. Each image produced is a narrative, a story about health, illness, healing and sometimes mystery.

At the heart of this world are the radiologists, those medical detectives, and the radiology nurses, those benevolent guardians of the patient. They are the interpreters of these visual narratives, translating every shadow, every nuance, every contrast into a language that the rest of the medical world can understand and use.

But beyond technique, radiology is also an art. You need a sharp eye to see the subtleties, a deft hand to guide the instruments, and a compassionate heart to support and reassure the patient during the examination. It's a delicate dance between machine and man, between technology and empathy.

So the next time you hear the word "radiology", think of this astonishing universe where the invisible is revealed, where every image is a story, and where science mingles with humanity to better understand and treat. Radiology is not just a medical speciality, it's a window onto the inner miracle of life.

How to use this book:
A guide for budding professionals

Entering the world of radiology, with its technical jargon, imposing machines and strict protocols, can seem daunting. But don't worry, you have in your hands the ideal tool for navigating this sea of information with confidence. Here are a few tips on how to use this book to the best of its ability and maximise your learning.

1. Start at the beginning.
Although it may seem obvious, it's essential to start with the basics. Familiarise yourself with the history of radiology, the main concepts and the fundamentals. This will provide you with a solid foundation on which to build your knowledge.

2. Don't rush your reading.
Radiology is a complex discipline, and each chapter of this book is designed to delve into a specific facet. Take the time to digest each section, reread if necessary, and above all, apply what you learn in your working environment.

3. Use the case studies.
Throughout the book, you will find real case studies that highlight concrete situations encountered in the world of radiology. These studies are not simply anecdotes, but learning tools. Analyse them, discuss them with your colleagues and use them as a starting point for reflection and debate.

4. Practice independent thinking.
Each chapter ends with a series of questions and reflections. Don't neglect them. Take a moment to answer, to question yourself, to fully integrate the content. These moments of personal reflection will strengthen your understanding.

5. Collaborate and share.
Radiology, like any medical discipline, is a team effort. Share what you learn with your colleagues, ask questions, form study groups. Surrounding yourself with like-minded people will enrich your learning experience.

6. Come back often.
This book is not designed to be read once and then put on a shelf. As you progress in your career, you'll find that some sections become more relevant, others need re-reading. Keep it handy and use it as an ongoing resource.

7. Get actively involved.
The best way to learn is to do. Put your knowledge into

practice, get involved in research projects, attend conferences and constantly seek to broaden your horizons.

This book is more than just a source of information. It's a companion, a paper mentor, designed to guide you at every stage of your radiology career. Every page is an invitation to discover, every chapter a step closer to professional excellence. So, dear budding professionals, open your eyes wide, immerse yourself in this treasure trove of knowledge, and get ready to illuminate the invisible world of radiology.

Chapter 1:
DIVING INTO THE UNIVERSE
RADIOLOGY

History of radiology : From X-rays to MRI

Radiology occupies a unique place in the great saga of medicine. It is a story of innovation, accidental discoveries, daring pioneers, and the constant evolution of our ability to see beyond the surface. From the discovery of X-rays to the advent of MRI, embark on a fascinating journey through time.

In the beginning were X-rays

In 1895, Wilhelm Conrad Röntgen, a German physicist, made a discovery that was to revolutionise the world of medicine. While experimenting with cathode ray tubes, he noticed a fluorescent glow coming from a nearby screen. Intrigued, he continued his investigations and discovered X-rays, capable of penetrating matter and producing images on a photographic plate. The most famous image from this period is that of his wife's hand, clearly showing the bones. Radiology was born.

The First World War: battlefield and ground for innovation

During the Great War, the need to quickly locate bullets and shrapnel in soldiers' bodies made radiology an essential medical tool. The "Little Curies", mobile radiography units, were deployed at the front, marking a crucial stage in the recognition of the importance of radiology in patient care.

The post-war years: expansion and specialisation

The decades that followed saw exponential growth in the use of X-rays in medicine. Equipment became more sophisticated, allowing better quality images. Fluoroscopy made its appearance, offering images in real time.

The advent of tomography

In the 1970s, computerised axial tomography (CT) revolutionised radiology. Thanks to the use of computers, it was now possible to obtain three-dimensional images of the body, providing previously unequalled detail.

The era of MRI

The next decade saw the introduction of Magnetic Resonance Imaging (MRI). Instead of X-rays, MRI uses magnetic fields and radio waves to produce detailed images, particularly of soft tissue. Its ability to visualise the brain and other internal organs with exceptional precision has made it an invaluable tool.

Looking to the future: innovation and new horizons

Today, radiology continues to evolve at a breathtaking pace. New techniques, such as functional magnetic resonance imaging (fMRI) and positron emission tomography (PET), are opening up new horizons in the understanding and treatment of disease.

Looking back, the trajectory of radiology is truly astonishing. From its humble beginnings with X-rays to today's cutting-edge technology, it reflects our relentless quest to understand the human body, to see the invisible, and to provide better, more effective care for all. The history of radiology is living testimony to humanity's ability to innovate and transcend its limits. And who knows what the future will bring?

The radiology nurse :
Role, responsibilities and a typical day

The radiology nurse is often the hidden soul of the department, providing an essential link between technology and the patient. Her mission is more than just administering conventional nursing care. She is at the heart of an advanced technological environment, and her role requires as much clinical skill as humanity.

The role of the radiology nurse
In the world of radiology, the nurse is a central pivot. She prepares the patient for the examination, ensures his comfort, sometimes manages the contrast products, monitors his health during the procedure and looks after him on discharge. She also acts as an intermediary between the patient and the radiologist, translating complex information into simple terms to reassure and inform the patient.

Key responsibilities

- **Preparing the patient:** The nurse takes a medical history, checks that the patient has no contraindications to the examination, and explains the forthcoming procedure.
- **Management of contrast agents:** Some X-rays require the use of contrast agents. The nurse checks for allergies, sometimes prepares and administers these products, and monitors any reactions.
- **Continuous monitoring:** During the examination, the nurse monitors the patient's vital signs and intervenes in the event of any abnormality or discomfort.
- **Post-examination care:** After the examination, the nurse makes sure that the patient is feeling well, gives post-care advice if necessary, and prepares him or her for departure.

A typical day for a radiology nurse
8:00 - Arrival and inspection of the radiology room. Check equipment and prepare supplies for the day.
8.30am - First patient seen. Pre-examination interview, preparation and setting up for radiography.

9.15am - Administration of a contrast agent for a CT scan. Patient monitoring during the examination.

10:00 - Management of an anxious patient. Discussion, reassurance and building confidence before the MRI scan.

11:30 - Quick lunch break.

12:00 - Assistance during an interventional procedure, such as an X-ray-guided biopsy.

13:30 - Post-examination care for several patients.

2.15pm - Continuing education: learning a new technique or piece of equipment with the team.

3.00 pm - Accompanying a child for an X-ray. Use of distraction techniques to facilitate the examination.

16:30 - Last patients of the day.

17:00 - Cleaning and disinfecting the room. Preparation for the next day.

17:30 - Departure.

Above and beyond these tasks, what really sets radiology nurses apart is their ability to combine technical expertise with human competence. Every patient is unique, with their own concerns and needs, and the nurse is there to make their experience as pleasant as possible. In a world where machines are omnipresent, the human being remains at the centre of everything. And that's where the radiology nurse really shines.

The language of radiology : Glossary of terms and essential abbreviations

Radiology has its own jargon, a mixture of technical expressions, medical terms and abbreviations. For radiology nurses, mastering this language is essential. Here's a look at some of the key terms and abbreviations used in everyday radiology work.

Key terms :

 Radiography: Medical imaging technique using X-rays to visualise the inside of the body, particularly the bones.

 Scanner (or CT): Computerised axial tomography. Imaging technique producing three-dimensional images of the body.

 MRI: Magnetic Resonance Imaging. Technique using magnetic fields to obtain detailed images of soft tissue.

 Fluoroscopy: A technique that uses X-rays to visualise internal structures in real time.

 Contrast product: Substance administered to the patient to improve the visibility of certain structures or fluids during imaging.

 Guided biopsy: tissue sample taken with the help of an imaging technique to precisely target the area concerned.

Common abbreviations :

 AP: Antero-posterior (direction in which X-rays pass through the body).

 PA: Posteroanterior (opposite of AP).

 LL: Left flanker (side view, left side).

 RL: Right lateral (side view, right side).

 DV: Dorso-ventral (back to belly).

 VD: Ventro-dorsal (belly to back).

 TDM: Tomodensitométrie (French equivalent of CT scan).

 FOV: Field of View in MRI.

 PACS: Picture Archiving and Communication System.

 TE: Echo time (MRI parameter).

 TR: Repetition time (another MRI parameter).

It is important to note that the above list is not exhaustive and that radiology is a constantly evolving field. New terms and abbreviations are regularly introduced with the advent of new technologies and techniques.

Mastering this lexicon enables the radiology nurse to communicate effectively with the medical team, to understand the specific demands and needs of examinations, and to explain procedures to patients clearly. It's the key to navigating the fascinating but sometimes confusing world of radiology with confidence.

Chapter 2:
SAFETY FIRST

The principles of radiation protection: Why is it important?

In the glittering world of radiology, radiation protection is the silent sentinel. It ensures that the miracle of seeing through the human body does not turn into a curse for those who work in it, or for the patients who benefit from it. Understanding the importance of radiation protection is vital for any professional working in this field, especially radiology nurses, who are often the first point of contact for patients.

The essence of radiation protection :
Radiation protection, as its name suggests, aims to protect against the harmful effects of ionising radiation. Although this radiation is beneficial for diagnosis and certain treatments, it can have deleterious effects on biological tissues.
Why it's crucial:

- **Patient protection:** Incorrect dosing or unnecessary exposure to radiation can increase the risk of long-term cell damage or cancer.
- **Protection of personnel:** Health professionals are at risk because they are regularly in close proximity to sources of radiation. Adequate protection and training reduce this risk.
- **Legal and ethical responsibility:** Radiation protection standards are governed by laws and directives. Neglecting them can have legal and ethical consequences.

The three fundamental principles of radiation protection :

Justification: Any medical procedure involving exposure to radiation must be justified. This means that the expected benefits for the patient must outweigh the potential risks.

Optimisation: Exposure must be as low as reasonably achievable (ALARA principle - "As Low As Reasonably Achievable"). This means using as little radiation as possible to obtain the required image, optimising machine settings and using protective equipment.

Dose limits: Exposure limits have been set to ensure that no one, neither patient nor professional, is exposed to dangerous levels of radiation.

The day-to-day reality of radiation protection :

Radiation protection is more than just a matter of principle; it is a practical reality in the day-to-day work of a radiology nurse. She wears a lead apron to protect herself during procedures, stands behind protective screens whenever possible, wears a dosimeter to monitor her personal exposure, and guides patients to ensure that they are correctly positioned and protected.

Radiation protection is a delicate balancing act between medical necessity, protection and responsibility. It requires constant vigilance and ongoing training. But, ultimately, it ensures that radiology, that magic window on the invisible, remains a blessing rather than a threat to humanity.

Safety measures
for healthcare professionals

Despite its many diagnostic and therapeutic advantages, radiology presents risks inherent in ionising radiation. Health professionals working in this field are therefore exposed to these dangers. Ensuring their safety is an absolute priority. This requires not only knowledge, but also a set of preventive measures and concrete actions.

1. Understanding the risks :
First and foremost, a thorough understanding of the dangers associated with ionising radiation is essential. Regular training on the risks, their consequences and how to prevent them is an essential starting point.

2. Personal dosimetry :

   Dosimeter: Each professional is equipped with a personal dosimeter that measures cumulative exposure to radiation. These dosimeters are regularly analysed to ensure that exposure remains within acceptable limits.

   Regular monitoring: Dosimeter readings are carefully monitored and action is taken if an individual approaches exposure limits.

3. Use of protective equipment :

   Lead aprons: These aprons, often worn during X-ray examinations, protect against direct exposure.

   Thyroid collars: These protect the thyroid gland, which is particularly sensitive to radiation.

   Leaded goggles: To protect the eyes, another sensitive area.

   Protective screens: In examination rooms, leaded screens or partitions are often used to protect staff who must not be in the immediate vicinity of the patient.

4. Distancing and positioning :

   Keep as far away as possible from the source of radiation when on duty, respecting the inverse square rule: doubling the distance reduces exposure by a factor of four.

   Use remote imaging techniques or automation where available.

5. Minimising exposure time :
    Reduce the time spent close to the source of radiation.
    Plan procedures to minimise unnecessary exposure.
6. Optimising radiology equipment :
    Regular maintenance of equipment to ensure it is in good working order.
    Ongoing training in the use of the machines to ensure that the doses administered are as low as possible while maintaining optimum image quality.
7. Emergency protocols :
    To have clear protocols in place in the event of radiological incidents or accidents, to ensure a rapid and effective response.
8. Safe working environment :
    Design of radiology rooms to maximise protection: sealed walls, light signals indicating when equipment is in operation, clearly defined areas for staff and patients.
9. Awareness and communication :
    Encouraging open dialogue within the team on best practice, safety concerns and innovations.
    Promote a safety culture in which every member feels responsible for protecting everyone else.

In short, safety in radiology is a combination of knowledge, preparation, equipment and culture. Every radiology healthcare professional is the guardian of both their own safety and that of their colleagues. By adopting and respecting these measures, they ensure that radiology remains a powerful tool for patient care, while preserving their own well-being.

Precautions for patients:
Pregnancy, children and special cases

Radiology, in its various applications, is an invaluable diagnostic and therapeutic tool. However, certain populations, because of their vulnerability, require special attention. Ensuring their safety and well-being requires in-depth understanding and appropriate measures.

Pregnancy:
Pregnancy is a crucial time when exposure to ionising radiation must be minimised, as the foetus is particularly sensitive.

Communication: It is essential to inform healthcare professionals of any possibility of pregnancy before a radiological examination.

Benefit-risk assessment: If an examination is required, a careful assessment of the benefits against the potential risks is carried out.

Alternative techniques: Where possible, non-ionising imaging methods such as ultrasound or MRI are considered.

Targeted protection: If an X-ray examination is essential, specific protection for the abdomen is used to minimise foetal exposure.

Children:
Because of their rapid growth and long life expectancy, children are at greater risk of long-term effects from radiation.

Appropriate dosage: The equipment is adjusted to administer the lowest possible dose while guaranteeing a quality image.

Restricting examinations: Only examinations that are absolutely necessary are carried out.

Protection and restraint: Specific protection is used, and gentle restraint techniques can be employed to prevent the child from moving during the examination.

Support: When it is safe to do so, a parent or guardian can be present to reassure the child.

Special cases :

There are many other scenarios that require special precautions.

Patients with implantable devices: People with pacemakers, insulin pumps or other implantable electronic devices should be assessed before certain examinations, particularly MRI, because of the risk of interference.

Allergies : Before contrast products are administered, it is essential to assess the patient's allergy history.

Renal impairment: Some contrast media may affect renal function. Prior assessment is necessary for these patients.

Patients with reduced mobility: adapted equipment and techniques are used to facilitate their experience during examinations.

The essence of these precautions is to ensure patient safety while maximising the diagnostic or therapeutic benefits of radiology. Every patient is unique, and an individualised approach, based on effective communication and a thorough understanding of risks, will ensure the highest quality of care.

Chapter 3:
EQUIPMENT
AND TECHNOLOGIES EMPLOYED

Understanding the different types of imaging: X-ray, CT, MRI, ultrasound, etc.

Radiology encompasses a multitude of imaging techniques, each with its own specific features, advantages and indications. For healthcare professionals, and particularly for radiology nurses, understanding these different modalities is essential to ensuring optimal care.

1. X-ray :
   - **Principle:** Radiography uses X-rays, a form of ionising radiation, to produce two-dimensional images.
   - **Use:** Very common for visualising bones, lungs, heart and other organs.
   - **Advantages:** Fast, easily accessible and relatively inexpensive.
   - **Precautions: Because** of the radiation involved, adequate protection is essential.
2. Computed tomography (CT or scanner) :
   - **Principle:** The scanner also uses X-rays, but it captures a series of images from different angles to produce three-dimensional or 'slice' images of the body.
   - **Use:** Searching for tumours, bleeding, wounds, etc.
   - **Benefits:** Provides detailed images of soft tissue, bone and blood vessels.
   - **Precautions :** More radiation than standard radiography.

3. Magnetic resonance imaging (MRI) :
  Principle: Uses a powerful magnetic field and radio waves to obtain images of the body.
  Applications: Examines the brain, spinal cord, joints and other soft tissues.
  Advantages: No ionising radiation and extremely detailed images.
  Precautions: Patients with metallic or electronic devices must be assessed prior to the examination.
4. Ultrasound :
  Principle: Uses sound waves to produce images of the body.
  Use: Commonly used to examine the foetus during pregnancy, as well as the heart, blood vessels, thyroid, etc.
  Advantages: Safe, non-invasive and without ionising radiation.
  Precautions: Depends very much on the skill of the operator.
5. Nuclear medicine :
  Principle: Patients receive a small quantity of radioactive material, which emits gamma rays captured by a special camera.
  Applications: Evaluating organ function, detecting certain forms of cancer.
  Advantages: Allows biological functions to be observed.
  Precautions: Requires injection of a radiotracer.
6. Angiography :
  Principle: Imaging technique using a contrast medium to visualise blood vessels.
  Use: To search for vascular anomalies, such as aneurysms or obstructions.
  Benefits: Clear images of vessels.
  Precautions : Use of X-rays, need to insert a catheter.

7. Bone densitometry (DXA) :
  - **Principle:** Measures bone mineral density to assess bone strength.
  - **Uses:** Diagnosis of osteoporosis.
  - **Benefits:** Quick and easy.
  - **Precautions:** Use a low dose of X-rays.

Each of these imaging modalities has its place in the diagnostic and therapeutic landscape. The choice of technique will depend on the medical condition, the advantages and disadvantages of each method, and the specific needs of the patient. An in-depth knowledge of these tools will enable healthcare professionals to optimise care and ensure patient safety and comfort.

Daily maintenance and checks: The importance operational equipment

Radiology is a medical world where technology reigns supreme. From simple X-rays to complex MRIs, each machine is a masterpiece of engineering, combining physics, electronics and computers to produce images of the human body. However, like all complex equipment, these machines require regular maintenance to keep them running at peak performance. That's why daily maintenance and checks are essential.

A safety issue:
First and foremost, the issue is one of safety. Faulty X-ray equipment can put patients and staff at risk, whether through excessive exposure to radiation, diagnostic errors due to poor-quality images, or physical accidents linked to mechanical malfunctions.

Reliable diagnosis :
Image quality is at the heart of radiology. A poorly maintained machine can produce blurred, discoloured or

distorted images, which can lead to incorrect diagnoses. Regular maintenance guarantees the accuracy and clarity of images, which are essential for a correct diagnosis.

Equipment durability:
X-ray machines represent a considerable financial investment for healthcare establishments. Ensuring their maintenance means guaranteeing their longevity and maximising the return on their investment. What's more, an unexpected breakdown can have serious consequences, both in financial terms and in terms of planning and patient care.

Legal responsibility and standards :
Radiology equipment is subject to strict standards set by regulatory authorities. Failure to comply with these standards, even unintentionally, can result in severe legal penalties. Daily checks and regular maintenance ensure that the equipment complies with these standards.

How to guarantee operational equipment :

- **Daily checks:** Before each session starts, it's essential to carry out a series of routine tests to make sure everything is working properly.
- **Preventive maintenance programmes: In** addition to daily checks, the equipment must undergo regular inspections by specialist technicians to ensure that it is working properly.
- **Ongoing training:** Staff must be trained not only in the use of the equipment, but also in the detection of warning signals indicating a potential problem.
- **Documentation:** Keeping a detailed record of all interventions, maintenance and checks is essential to ensure traceability and meet compliance standards.

Daily maintenance and checks on radiology equipment are far more than just a box to tick. It's an imperative to ensure patient safety, quality of care, equipment durability and compliance with standards. For the radiology nurse, having an operational machine means having a reliable ally in the daily battle for patient health.

Recent innovations and the technological future of radiology

Since its birth with the discovery of X-rays by Wilhelm Conrad Röntgen in 1895, radiology has never ceased to evolve, drawing on technological advances to push back the boundaries of medical imaging. While every decade has brought its share of revolutions, the last few years have been particularly rich in innovation. Let's take a look at recent advances and take a look at the promising future of radiology.

1. Digital radiology :
Although the switch from analogue to digital radiology is not an extremely recent innovation, its widespread adoption has transformed the way images are captured, stored and shared. Digital images offer better quality, are easier to archive and can be shared instantly around the world.

2. Artificial Intelligence (AI):
AI is undoubtedly the most significant technological revolution in radiology in recent years. It enables:

- **Image analysis:** AI can help identify anomalies on X-rays, CT scans or MRIs, often with the same or greater accuracy than humans.
- **Workflow management:** AI can optimise schedules, sort cases according to urgency, and improve patient management.

3. Radiomics :
Radiomics aims to extract a vast amount of information from medical images, far beyond what the human eye can perceive. This data can be used to better understand

34

diseases, predict their evolution and personalise treatments.

4. Hybrid imaging :
Combining different imaging modalities, such as PET-CT or PET-MRI, provides both functional and anatomical information. This multi-modal approach offers a more comprehensive view of pathologies.

5. Advances in MRI :
Techniques such as functional MRI (fMRI), which measures and maps brain activity, and diffusion MRI, which assesses tissue structure, are opening up new horizons in neuroimaging and oncology.

6. Augmented and virtual reality:
These technologies offer the possibility of superimposing radiological images on the surgeon's actual field during an operation, thus guiding the surgery with unrivalled precision.

The future of technology :

- **Miniaturisation:** The future could see increasingly compact devices, making medical imaging accessible even in remote areas.
- **Non-invasive techniques:** The aim is to reduce or even eliminate exposure to ionising radiation.
- **Interconnection of equipment:** In the age of "everything-connected", radiology equipment could be integrated into wider networks to improve the coordination of care.

Innovation in radiology is not just about technology. It's an ongoing quest to improve patient care, push back the boundaries of what we can 'see' and 'understand' about the human body, and transform the diagnosis and treatment of disease. For healthcare professionals, keeping abreast of these developments is essential to providing the best possible care.

Chapter 4:
PATIENT PREPARATION
AND PROCEDURES

Patient intake and assessment :
First impressions count

The first meeting between a patient and the radiology nurse is much more than a simple formality. It's a crucial stage that lays the foundations for a relationship of trust between patient and healthcare professional. From the warm welcome to the preliminary assessment, every detail counts. In the world of radiology, where patients can be anxious about impressive machines and uncertain diagnoses, first impressions are all the more important.

1. The importance of a warm welcome :
A smile, a handshake, a clear introduction: these simple gestures create a climate of trust. Patients should feel recognised, respected and safe from the moment they enter the radiology department. The humanity behind the professional mask is essential to reassure and reassure the patient.

2. Communication: the key to successful evaluation :
   Active listening: The nurse must be attentive to the patient's concerns, questions and feelings. Listening is a valuable tool for understanding the patient's expectations and identifying any concerns.

   Open questions: Rather than asking closed questions requiring "yes" or "no" answers, the nurse should encourage the patient to share more by asking open-ended questions.

3. Clear explanation of procedures :
The unknown is often a source of anxiety. By clearly

explaining what the patient can expect, the nurse demystifies the process and reduces apprehension. Explanatory brochures or videos can also be useful.

4. Preliminary medical assessment :

Prior to any radiological examination, a preliminary assessment is required to ensure that the patient is fit to undergo the procedure. This includes:

Medical history: Any relevant history, such as recent surgery, allergies or potential pregnancy, should be identified.

Contraindications: For some procedures, contraindications may exist, such as the presence of metal implants for an MRI scan.

5. Managing patient anxiety :

It is not uncommon for patients to feel anxious before a radiological examination. A few strategies can help:

Relaxation techniques: Patients can be taught simple breathing or visualisation techniques to help them relax.

Create a soothing environment: A pleasant waiting room, soft music or relaxing images can help to relax the atmosphere.

6. Confidentiality and dignity :

Respect for confidentiality is essential. The nurse must ensure that medical information is treated with the utmost care and that the patient feels comfortable and respected throughout the procedure.

Welcoming and assessing radiology patients are delicate moments that require finesse, empathy and professionalism. The first impression, as they say, is the one that sticks. For the radiology nurse, this is a unique opportunity to establish a relationship of trust, reassure the patient and ensure that the examination goes smoothly.

Preparation for various exams: What every nurse needs to know

Radiology is a vast and varied field, encompassing a multitude of examinations ranging from standard radiography to advanced MRI. Proper preparation of the patient is essential to ensure not only patient safety but also image quality. Here's what every radiology nurse needs to know to best prepare their patients for different types of examination.

1. Standard radiography (X-ray) :
   - **Clothing preparation:** The patient must remove any jewellery, glasses or metal objects that could interfere with the image.
   - **Positioning:** Particular attention must be paid to positioning the patient to obtain the best possible image.
2. Computed tomography (CT or scanner) :
   - **Fasting:** If a contrast medium is to be used, the patient may have to fast for several hours before the examination.
   - **Allergies: It** is vital to check whether the patient has any allergies, particularly to iodine, which is used in certain contrast products.
   - **Hydration:** Encouraging the patient to drink water can help eliminate the contrast medium after the examination.
3. Magnetic resonance imaging (MRI) :
   - **Safety: It** is vital to ensure that the patient has no metal implants or other devices that could be affected by the magnetic field.
   - **Anxiety:** MRI can be noisy and confining, so it's important to prepare patients for the experience and offer support if they feel anxious.

4. Ultrasound :
   Specific preparation: Depending on the area of the body to be examined, the patient may need to drink water or fast.
   Appropriate clothing: It is preferable to wear clothing that is easy to remove or raise to facilitate access to the area to be examined.
5. Interventional radiography and angiography :
   Fasting: Patients often have to fast before the procedure.
   Informed consent: Before any interventional procedure, it is essential to obtain the patient's consent after explaining the risks and benefits.
6. Mammography :
   Avoid deodorants: Certain deodorants or powders can interfere with image quality. It is therefore advisable to avoid wearing them on the day of the examination.
   Emotional preparation: This examination can be uncomfortable and anxiety-provoking for some women, so emotional support and clear communication are essential.
7. Scintigraphy and PET scan :
   Medication: Certain medications can affect the result of the examination. It is therefore important to check the patient's list of treatments.
   Fasting: Fasting is often required before these examinations.

Proper preparation of the patient is essential to ensure the success of each radiological examination. In addition to their technical skills, radiology nurses must be good listeners, good teachers and adaptable to the specific needs of each patient and each examination.

Pain and stress management: The humanity behind every image

Beyond its technological advances, radiology is an art that combines science and humanity. Patients who walk through the doors of a radiology department carry with them much more than just physical symptoms. Fear, anxiety, apprehension, sometimes even pain, are all emotions and sensations that need to be taken into account. This is where the nurse comes in, not only as a health professional, but also as an emotional and human support.

1. Recognising pain :
   - **Objective assessment:** Use pain scales to quantify the patient's level of pain.
   - **Active listening:** Pain is subjective, and the patient's description is essential for an accurate assessment.
2. Non-pharmacological techniques :
   - **Distraction:** Offer music, videos or even VR goggles to entertain the patient during the procedure.
   - **Deep breathing and relaxation techniques:** Simple techniques can help reduce anxiety and pain.
3. Pharmacological approach :
   - **Administration of analgesics:** Depending on the level of pain and the patient's history.
   - **Sedation:** In specific cases, light sedation may be considered to ensure patient comfort.
4. Managing stress and anxiety :
   - **Psychological preparation:** Clearly explaining the forthcoming procedure can often defuse many fears.
   - **A reassuring presence: The** nurse's simple presence, attentiveness and caring touch can greatly reduce stress levels.

5. Continuing education :

   Keeping up to date: Pain management is a constantly evolving field. Nurses need to keep abreast of new techniques and approaches.

   Exchanges with colleagues: Sharing experiences and tips with your peers enriches your practices.

6. The importance of follow-up :

   After the procedure: Always check how the patient is feeling. A debriefing may sometimes be necessary, particularly if the patient did not enjoy the examination.

   Feedback: Encourage patients to share their experiences in order to continually improve the service.

Although radiology is centred on imaging, it must above all remain a patient-centred practice. Each image tells the story of an individual, with their fears, hopes and sometimes their pain. As a radiology nurse, recognising and managing these elements is just as essential as mastering the technical aspects of the profession. It is this alchemy of skill and compassion that makes the profession so rich.

Chapter 5:
EMERGENCIES AND UNFORESEEN EVENTS

Reacting to allergic reactions and medical emergencies

Radiology, while primarily a diagnostic field, is not without risks. The possibility of an allergic reaction to contrast agents, malaise or other medical emergencies requires adequate preparation on the part of the team, particularly the nurse, who is often the first line of response in the event of a complication.

1. Understanding the agents involved :
   - **Contrast products:** Although rare, allergic reactions can occur. It is essential to be aware of the signs of an allergic reaction, whether minor (skin rashes, itching) or major (anaphylactic shock).
   - **Other drugs :** Some patients may have unexpected reactions to other drugs used in radiology.
2. Pre-examination assessment :
   - **Medical history:** Systematically ask the patient about any known allergies and history of reactions to contrast products or drugs.
   - **Appropriate preparation:** In some cases, antihistamine premedication may be considered.
3. Rapid recognition of signs :
   - **Observation:** Watch for signs of respiratory distress, skin rash, changes in skin colour and any alteration in consciousness.
   - **Listen:** Patient complaints such as itching or burning may be the first signs of a reaction.

4. Intervention protocol :
   Alert: Notify the radiologist and medical team immediately.
   First aid: Depending on the severity, this may range from the administration of an antihistamine to resuscitation measures, such as the administration of adrenaline in the event of anaphylactic shock.
   Tools at hand: Always have a well-equipped and easily accessible emergency trolley containing emergency medicines, resuscitation equipment and a defibrillator.
5. After the emergency :
   Monitoring: Following a reaction, the patient should be closely monitored until stable.
   Documentation: All incidents must be meticulously documented in the patient's medical file.
   Debriefing: Bringing the team together to discuss the incident, evaluate the response and see if there are any areas for improvement.
6. Further training :
   Regular updates: Recommendations and protocols may evolve. Nurses must ensure that they keep up to date with best practice.
   Emergency simulations: Organise regular emergency simulations to ensure that the whole team is prepared to react quickly and effectively.

Every second counts in a medical emergency. For the radiology nurse, the ability to react quickly and appropriately can make the difference between a benign outcome and a potentially tragic situation. The importance of regular training, a well-prepared team and constant vigilance cannot be underestimated.

Managing trauma cases and radiological emergencies

Emergency radiology is an area where every minute can be crucial. Patients suffering trauma or other emergency situations often require rapid imaging to assess the extent of injuries and guide management. The nurse plays a central role here, acting as a link between the patient, the emergency medical team and the radiologist.

1. Rapid assessment :

   Triage: Distinguishing between cases requiring immediate intervention and other less urgent cases.

   Communication with the emergency doctor: Quickly understand the needs and priorities of each patient.

2. Preparing the patient :

   Stabilisation: In some cases, emergency measures (such as immobilisation) may be necessary before imaging.

   Essential information: quickly retrieve relevant information (type of trauma, areas of pain, medical history).

3. Choice of imaging modality :

   Standard X-ray: Often the first step in assessing fractures or other bone lesions.

   CT (computed tomography): Used for detailed assessment of trauma, particularly cranial, thoracic or abdominal.

   MRI: Less common in emergency situations, but can be used for specific lesions, particularly neurological lesions.

4. During the examination :

   Safety: Ensure that the patient is safe throughout the examination, particularly if unconscious or confused.

Monitoring: Monitor the patient's vital signs and pain, and be ready to intervene if their condition changes.
5. After the examination :
  Patient transfer: Depending on the results, the patient may require surgery, hospitalisation or other care.
  Communication: Transmit the results to the emergency doctor or surgeon in a concise and clear manner.
6. In the event of a radiological emergency :
  Contamination: In the event of a radiological emergency (such as accidental exposure to radiation), it is essential to follow decontamination protocols and ensure everyone's safety.
  Collaboration with experts: In the event of a radiological incident, close collaboration with medical physicists and radiation protection experts is crucial.
7. Continuing education and simulations :
  Regular training: Ensure that all teams are trained to respond effectively to emergencies and are familiar with the protocols.
  Emergency simulations: organising simulated situations to test and improve responses in real time.

Managing trauma cases and radiological emergencies requires the ability to act quickly and effectively while maintaining patient safety and well-being. Radiology nurses are often on the front line of this management and must possess a unique blend of technical and human skills to meet the challenges of these situations.

Importance of continuing training and emergency simulations

In the ever-changing world of radiology, the nurse's role extends beyond simply carrying out procedures to include a range of responsibilities that require regular updating of knowledge and skills. What's more, in an emergency context, proper preparation can literally mean the difference between life and death.

1. A profession in constant evolution :
   - **Emerging technologies :** With the advent of new imaging modalities and innovative techniques, it's essential to keep up to date to offer the best possible care.
   - **New methodologies:** Protocols and methods change as research advances, ensuring safer and more effective care.
2. Simulation as a learning tool :
   - **Scenarios:** Simulations provide a safe environment for practising emergency situations, without risk to patients.
   - **Feedback:** After a simulation, feedback is used to better understand errors, adjust techniques and improve future response.
3. Radiation protection :
   - **Latest recommendations:** As research develops, new recommendations for radiation protection may emerge.
   - **Best practice:** Ongoing training ensures that the nurse always uses the least radiation-intensive techniques possible, while obtaining high-quality images.
4. The importance of soft skills :
   - **Communication:** Knowing how and when to communicate effectively, particularly in stressful situations, is an essential skill.
   - **Teamwork:** Emergency simulations can help to strengthen team cohesion and improve inter-professional collaboration.

5. Preparing for rare but critical situations :
- **Severe allergic reactions, complications:** While these situations are rare, an inadequate response can have serious consequences. Simulations help to ensure a rapid and appropriate response.
- **Specific cases:** For example, how to manage a paediatric patient in crisis, or how to respond to a radiological accident.

6. Promoting the profession :
- **Professional recognition:** Commitment to ongoing training demonstrates professional excellence.
- **Assurance for the patient:** Patients are reassured in the knowledge that their nurse is regularly trained and prepared for emergencies.

Continuing education and emergency simulations are not simply supplements to a radiology nurse's initial training. They are essential elements in guaranteeing the safety, efficiency and excellence of the care provided. In an increasingly complex and specialised medical world, keeping up to date and practising regularly is becoming an absolute necessity if we are to offer the best to every patient.

Chapter 6:
TECHNOLOGICAL ADVANCES
AND RESEARCH

The latest innovations in medical imaging

Medical imaging has always been at the cutting edge of technology, constantly pushing back the boundaries of what we can see and understand about the human body. Each advance offers new insights, improves diagnostic accuracy, reduces risks to patients and opens the way to new methods of treatment. Here's a look at recent innovations in this exciting field.

1. Advanced digital radiography :
   - **More sensitive sensors:** Reduced radiation doses needed to obtain a clear image.
   - **Enhanced image processing:** Advanced algorithms for better detail detection.
2. Spectral computed tomography (CT) :
   - **Enhanced detail:** By using multiple energy spectra, this technology can differentiate tissue more accurately, helping to distinguish blood from clots, for example.
3. High-field magnetic resonance imaging (MRI) :
   - **Increased resolution:** More powerful magnets allow more detailed visualisation of internal structures, particularly useful for the brain and joints.
   - **Real-time functional MRI:** Monitoring changes in brain activity almost in real time.
4. Portable ultrasound imaging :
   - **Compact devices:** Innovations have resulted in ultra-portable devices that can be used at the patient's bedside, in rural areas or during field operations.

5. Hybrid positron emission tomography (PET) :
   Combination with other techniques: Combining PET with CT or MRI offers combined metabolic and anatomical imaging for precise localisation of areas of activity.
6. Artificial intelligence and machine learning :
   Image interpretation: AI can help detect anomalies that the human eye might miss, and suggest possible diagnoses.
   Procedure optimisation: Using AI to adjust imaging parameters in real time, maximising quality while minimising radiation dose.
7. Interventional radiology :
   Image-guided treatments: Minimally invasive techniques to treat conditions such as tumours, aneurysms or vascular obstructions.
8. Molecular imaging :
   Beyond anatomy: Visualisation of biological processes on a molecular scale, enabling a deeper understanding of diseases and responses to treatment.

These innovations in medical imaging are transforming not only the way doctors see and understand the human body, but also how they diagnose and treat disease. The combination of advanced technologies, intelligent algorithms and extensive training ensures that medical imaging will continue to play a central role in patient care for years to come.

Taking part in clinical research: why and how?

Clinical research is one of the cornerstones of medical progress. It is the process by which new therapies, drugs, medical devices and procedures are tested and evaluated to ensure their safety and effectiveness. For radiology nurses, understanding clinical research and considering participating in it can enrich their professional practice.

1. Why take part in clinical research?

Improving patient care: Clinical research leads to new discoveries that can improve patient care and treatment outcomes.

Career development: Participation in research enables nurses to broaden their skills and specialise in cutting-edge areas.

Contribution to science: Clinical research is essential to the advancement of medicine. Participating in this process contributes to the advancement of science.

Professional reputation: Institutions that are actively involved in research are often regarded as leaders in their field.

2. Understanding clinical research :

Types of research: There are several types of research, including observational studies, clinical trials and interventional studies.

Research protocol: Each study is guided by a strict protocol detailing how it will be conducted.

Research ethics: All research involving human beings must be approved by an ethics committee to ensure that it is ethical and safe.

3. How can I get involved in clinical research?

Training and education: Specific training in clinical research is often required to understand the process and regulations.

Finding opportunities: Hospitals, universities and private companies often offer research opportunities.

Collaboration: Working closely with researchers, doctors and other healthcare professionals can open doors to research opportunities.

4. The role of radiology nurses in clinical research :
- **Patient recruitment:** Identify and approach patients who may be eligible for certain studies.
- **Data collection:** Ensure that all data is collected accurately and in accordance with the protocol.
- **Patient monitoring:** Ensure patients are safe and report any side effects or problems.
- **Patient education:** Informing patients about the study, its purpose and what it involves.

5. Challenges and rewards :
- **Challenges :** Clinical research can be demanding in terms of time and resources. It requires rigour and attention to detail.
- **Rewards: As** well as contributing to medical progress, research offers the opportunity to learn, specialise and collaborate with experts in the field.

Clinical research is a fascinating and essential area of medicine. For radiology nurses, embarking on this path can not only enrich their careers, but can also make a significant contribution to improving patient care and advancing science.

The future of radiology : Projects and aspirations

Radiology is at an exciting crossroads in its history. With the intersection of technology, biology and medicine, its future seems limitless. As we look to the future, let's take a look at the projects and aspirations that could shape the next era of radiology.

1. The omnipresence of artificial intelligence (AI) :
- **Assisted diagnosis:** AI can help radiologists identify subtle anomalies and predict pathological trends before they become obvious.

Optimised workflow: thanks to AI, radiology procedures can be accelerated, from image capture to interpretation and report generation.

2. Personalised radiology :

Adaptation to the patient: Imaging protocols individually adapted to the patient's needs and medical history.

Targeted therapies: Using images to guide personalised treatments, such as interventional radiology.

3. Hybrid imaging :

Combining different modalities: For example, combining PET and MRI to obtain anatomical and metabolic information in a single examination.

Radiation reduction: Thanks to hybrid techniques, it is possible to reduce the radiation dose while still obtaining high-quality images.

4. Wireless radiology :

Portable technologies: Lighter, wireless devices to facilitate mobility and access to imaging in hard-to-reach or remote areas.

Advanced teleradiology: remote image interpretation, enabling expert consultation almost anywhere in the world.

5. Advanced molecular imaging :

At cellular level: Visualising and understanding processes at cellular and molecular level, opening the door to new diagnostic and therapeutic methods.

6. Immersive training and education :

Virtual reality (VR) and augmented reality (AR): Using these technologies to train radiologists by immersing them in realistic scenarios.

Emergency simulations: real-time training to prepare professionals for radiological emergencies.

7. Multidisciplinary collaboration :
  - **Integrated imaging centres:** Areas where radiologists, oncologists, surgeons and other specialists can work closely together.
  - **Holistic approach:** Integrating the psychological and social aspects of patient care into radiological practice.

The future of radiology is bright, with technological advances that promise to transform the discipline. The projects and aspirations outlined above are just the tip of the iceberg. As technology evolves and our understanding of biology deepens, radiology will continue to play a vital role in the medical landscape, improving patient care and shaping the future of medicine.

Chapter 7:
RADIOLOGICAL EMERGENCIES AND ENVIRONMENTAL

Introduction to radiological emergencies: Types and causes

When we think of medical emergencies, the image that often springs to mind is that of a busy emergency room, with doctors and nurses bustling around patients presenting a multitude of symptoms. However, in the context of radiology, an emergency takes on a different dimension. It refers to situations requiring rapid medical imaging intervention to make a diagnosis, assess the extent of an injury or even guide treatment. Let's take a closer look at the types of radiological emergencies and their common causes.

1. Traumatic emergencies :
- **Fractures:** Bone fractures, whether simple or complex, often require an X-ray or CT scan to determine their severity and guide management.
- **Head injuries: In the** event of a head injury, a brain scan can be crucial in detecting haemorrhage, oedema or a skull fracture.
- **Thoracic and abdominal trauma:** Road accidents, falls or other injuries can cause damage to internal organs, requiring urgent imaging for assessment.

2. Non-traumatic emergencies :
- **Stroke (cerebrovascular accident): If a** stroke is suspected, a CT scan or MRI of the brain is necessary to determine whether it is an ischaemic or haemorrhagic stroke.

- **Intestinal obstruction:** Symptoms of intestinal obstruction may require urgent imaging to confirm the diagnosis and locate the site of obstruction.
- **Severe infection:** In some cases, radiology can be used to locate the source of a deep infection, such as an abscess.

3. Interventional emergencies :
- **Internal haemorrhage: In the case of** internal haemorrhage, interventional radiology can be used to locate the source of bleeding and perform embolisation.
- **Thrombosis:** Blood clots, such as those responsible for pulmonary embolism, may require radiological intervention to dissolve or remove them.

4. Causes of radiological emergencies :
- **Trauma:** Road accidents, falls, sports injuries or other forms of physical trauma may require emergency imaging.
- **Pathological changes:** Pre-existing illnesses or medical complications, such as infections or blood clots, may suddenly worsen.
- **Post-operative:** Following certain surgical procedures, complications may arise that require urgent radiological assessment.

Radiological emergencies cover a wide range of situations, from physical trauma to medical complications. In each case, rapid and accurate imaging is essential to guide treatment and improve patient outcomes. The ability to intervene quickly in emergency situations is one of the many essential skills of radiology professionals.

Managing a radiological emergency: Protocols and safety measures

When faced with a radiological emergency, the priority is to ensure patient safety while obtaining clear, accurate images to guide diagnosis or treatment. This requires a combination of strict protocols and safety measures to ensure the well-being of both patient and medical staff. Let's take a look at how these emergencies are managed.

1. Initial assessment of the patient :
    Triage: First of all, the patient is assessed by a medical team to determine the urgency and the type of imaging required.
    Medical history: It is essential to gather relevant information quickly, such as allergies, surgical history or the possibility of pregnancy.
2. Preparation for imaging :
    Positioning : Ensure patient comfort while obtaining the best angle for imaging.
    Protection against radiation : Use of lead shields or other protection for areas of the body not targeted by the examination.
3. Clear communication :
    Patient information: Briefly explain the procedure to the patient, reassuring them and answering any questions they may have.
    Team coordination: Effective communication between radiologists, technicians, nurses and referring physicians is essential for managing emergencies.
4. Safety measures during the examination :
    Monitoring: Constant monitoring of the patient during the examination, especially if the patient is in a critical situation.

- **Equipment settings:** Ensure that the equipment is set to minimise exposure to radiation while still obtaining high-quality images.

5. Fast, accurate interpretation :
- **Radiologist availability:** In emergency situations, the immediate availability of a radiologist to interpret images is crucial.
- **Transmission of results:** Results must be communicated quickly and clearly to the treating medical team for immediate action if necessary.

6. Post-imaging :
- **Follow-up:** Monitor the patient's condition after the examination, especially if contrast products have been used.
- **Documentation:** Accurately documenting the entire event, from imaging details to patient observations.

7. Prevention and training :
- **Simulations:** Organise regular emergency simulations to train and prepare staff to manage these situations.
- **Updating protocols:** Regularly review and update protocols in line with the latest research and recommendations.

Managing a radiological emergency requires both technical skill and human sensitivity. Every stage, from the initial assessment to the communication of results, must be carried out with care and speed. Protocols and safety measures are not just guidelines, but vital tools to ensure that, even in the most tense situations, every patient receives quality care.

Case studies :
Historical disasters and lessons learned

Over the years, a number of disasters, whether natural, industrial or accidental, have highlighted the challenges and needs of radiology in emergency situations. Let's take a look at some of these major disasters and the lessons they have taught us about radiology.

1. Chernobyl, 1986:
    - **Context:** The explosion and fire at the Chernobyl nuclear power plant released large quantities of radioactive materials into the atmosphere.
    - **Role of radiology:** Assessment and monitoring of workers and residents exposed to radiation.
    - **Lessons learned:** The importance of rapid intervention, radiation protection training and the need for equipment to assess radioactive contamination.
2. The Kobe earthquake, 1995 :
    - **Context:** A violent earthquake struck the Japanese city of Kobe, causing extensive damage and injuring thousands of people.
    - **Role of radiology:** management of casualties, detection of fractures and other internal injuries.
    - **Lessons learned:** The need for a mobile and resilient radiology infrastructure to respond in the event of a natural disaster.
3. The attacks of 11 September 2001 :
    - **Context:** Terrorist attacks have hit the United States, including the Twin Towers in New York.
    - **Role of radiology:** Management of trauma victims and coordination with other medical services.
    - **Lessons learned:** The importance of disaster preparedness and training radiologists to manage large-scale events.

4. The Fukushima nuclear disaster, 2011 :

    Context: Following a tsunami, the Fukushima nuclear power plant experienced several explosions, releasing radioactive materials.

    Role of radiology: Monitoring and assessment of radioactive contamination in residents and workers.

    Lessons learned: The need for clear protocols for evacuation, decontamination and communication with the public about radiological risks.

5. The earthquake in Haiti, 2010 :

    Context: A devastating earthquake has hit Haiti, causing enormous loss of life and property.

    Role of radiology: medical support for the injured, particularly for fractures, head injuries and thoracic trauma.

    Lessons learned: The need for portable radiology equipment, specific training and coordination with international humanitarian organisations.

Each of these disasters highlighted specific and crucial aspects of radiology in emergency situations. The lessons learned have shaped and improved radiologists' preparedness and response to such situations. Although these events were tragic, they also highlighted the importance and value of radiology in the management of large-scale emergencies and disasters.

Chapter 8:
RADIOPEDIATRICS :
SPECIFIC FEATURES AND CHALLENGES

The particularities of imaging in children

Medical imaging in children is a special field that requires a tailored approach, both in terms of imaging techniques and management of the young patient. Because of children's continuous growth and development, as well as their particular sensitivity to radiation, paediatric imaging requires specialist expertise.

1. Changing physiology and anatomy :
   - **Bone growth:** Children's bones are actively growing, with the presence of growth plate requiring special interpretation on imaging.
   - **Developing organs:** Children's organs, particularly the brain, continue to develop and have characteristics specific to each age.
2. Increased sensitivity to radiation :
   - **Minimum doses:** Children are more sensitive to the effects of radiation than adults. It is therefore crucial to minimise the radiation dose during X-ray examinations.
   - **Alternative techniques:** Whenever possible, it is preferable to use non-radiation imaging techniques such as ultrasound or MRI.
3. Different psychological approach :
   - **Communication:** Children need age-appropriate explanations to understand the procedure.
   - **Comfort and safety:** The examination room should be designed to reassure the child, with soothing visual and audio elements.

- **Parents' presence:** Allowing parents to accompany their child during the examination can be beneficial for the child's emotional comfort.

4. Specific imaging techniques :
- **Positioning:** Children may require specific positions or restraint devices to ensure quality images.
- **Contrast products:** The doses and types of contrast products must be adjusted for children.

5. Pathologies specific to childhood :
- **Congenital diseases:** Certain anomalies may be present from birth and require specific imaging to diagnose them.
- **Common paediatric conditions:** Conditions such as osteochondritis and Legg-Calvé-Perthes disease are specific to the paediatric population.

6. Collaboration with other specialists :
- **Multidisciplinary team:** Paediatric radiology often benefits from close collaboration with other specialists, such as paediatricians, paediatric surgeons and others.

Imaging children is a specific branch of radiology that requires not only technical mastery but also great sensitivity and adaptability. The priority is to guarantee the child's safety and comfort while obtaining accurate images for appropriate diagnosis and treatment.

Communication and reassurance young patients and their parents

In radiology, as in many other medical fields, communication is essential, especially when it comes to young patients and their parents. Imaging procedures can be stressful, even frightening, for a child, and their parents may also be worried. Here's how to approach communication in this particular context to reassure everyone.

1. Establishing a connection with the child :
    Appropriate language: Use simple, age-appropriate terms. For example, instead of "X-ray", you could say "photo of the inside".
    Involve the child: Ask them questions, ask them how they feel and encourage them to ask their own questions.
    Use analogies: For example, compare the scanner to a "big camera" or the MRI to a "space shuttle".
2. Involving parents :
    Explain the procedure: Tell the parents what's going to happen, how long the examination will take and how important it is to the diagnosis.
    Address concerns: Reassure them about the safety of procedures and discuss any specific precautions, such as radiation protection.
    Encourage attendance: If possible, and if it does not disrupt the examination, allow parents to be present during the procedure to reassure their child.
3. Create a reassuring environment :
    Appropriate decor: An examination room with bright colours or soothing images can help to relax the child.
    Distractions: Provide toys, books or even videos to help distract and calm the child before or during the exam.
    The right equipment: Use equipment that is the right size for your child so that they feel more comfortable.
4. Take your time :
    Don't rush: If a child is particularly anxious, it may be useful to give them a few extra minutes to familiarise themselves with the environment.
    Reassurance through touch: A simple gesture, such as a hand on the shoulder, can be very soothing.

5. After the examination :
- **Praise the child:** Thank them for their cooperation and tell them they've done well.
- **Post-examination discussion:** Talk to your parents about the results (insofar as you are authorised to do so) and what happens next, such as a possible follow-up consultation.

Effective communication is the key to ensuring a positive experience for young radiology patients. By understanding and responding to their emotional needs, as well as those of their parents, you can greatly improve comfort and cooperation during imaging procedures.

Specific cases: common pathologies and paediatric emergencies

Paediatric radiology presents a unique set of challenges due to the different pathologies and emergencies that are commonly encountered in children. This section focuses on the most common conditions that require radiological intervention, as well as how to deal effectively with these situations.

1. Bone and joint disorders :
- **Growth fractures:** The growth plate, or physis, is the area of developing bone that is particularly vulnerable to fracture in children.
- **Osteomyelitis:** An infection of the bone that may occur suddenly or slowly. Imaging can help identify the extent of the infection and guide treatment.
- **Legg-Calvé-Perthes disease:** A hip condition in which blood flow to the head of the femur is interrupted.

2. Thoracic disorders :

Pneumonia: A common lung infection in children which can be diagnosed by X-ray.

Foreign bodies: Children can aspirate small objects, requiring X-rays to locate and guide extraction.

3. Abdominal trauma :

Organ damage: Trauma such as falls or impacts can lead to organ damage. Imaging can help assess severity.

Appendicitis: An inflammation of the appendix, common in children, may require an ultrasound or CT scan to confirm the diagnosis.

4. Neurological disorders :

Meningitis: An inflammation of the membranes surrounding the brain and spinal cord. Although diagnosed clinically, an MRI scan may sometimes be necessary to assess complications.

Intracranial haemorrhage: Head injuries can lead to bleeding inside the skull, requiring urgent imaging.

5. Urogenital disorders :

Hydronephrosis: An enlargement of the kidney due to an obstruction in the flow of urine. Ultrasound is commonly used for diagnosis.

Testicular torsion: An emergency in which the testicle twists, cutting off its blood supply. Ultrasound is essential for rapid diagnosis.

6. Other emergencies :

Sepsis: A reaction by the body to a serious infection. Imaging can help identify the source of the infection.

Poisoning/Intoxication: Accidental ingestion of toxic substances may require imaging to assess the effects or locate the pills.

Paediatric radiology emergencies require the ability to react quickly and accurately. Knowledge of common pathologies and associated radiological signs is essential to ensure that these young patients are properly cared for. Specialist training and close collaboration with other paediatric specialists ensure that these children receive the best possible care.

Chapter 9:
ECOLOGY IN RADIOLOGY

Environmental impact
equipment and consumables

Despite its spectacular medical advances, radiology is not without impact on the environment. Imposing machines, considerable electricity consumption, specific waste... All these factors have ecological consequences. Here's a look at the environmental impact of radiology.

1. Manufacture of equipment :
   - **Resources extracted :** The production of sophisticated machines requires rare metals, plastics and other materials, the extraction of which can disrupt ecosystems.
   - **CO_2 emissions:** The manufacture of radiology equipment generates carbon emissions, particularly during the production of electronic components.
2. Energy consumption of equipment :
   - **Intensive use:** Equipment such as CT scanners and MRI scanners consume a lot of energy, especially when they are running almost continuously in large hospitals.
   - **Cooling requirements:** Some equipment, particularly MRI, requires cooling systems that also consume energy.
3. Waste and consumables :
   - **X-ray waste:** Traditional x-ray film contains chemicals that can be harmful if not disposed of correctly.
   - **Disposable consumables:** Items such as sheets, protective clothing and other items can generate a significant amount of waste.

4. End-of-life of equipment :
   Disposal: X-ray machines have a limited lifespan. Their disposal requires appropriate decontamination and recycling, which is not always carried out in the best possible way.
   Reuse and recycling: While some parts can be recycled, others, particularly electronic components, can end up in landfill, with an associated environmental impact.
5. Contrast products and drugs :
   Manufacturing: The production of contrast products requires resources and generates waste.
   Disposal: Once used, these products are often excreted by patients and can end up in wastewater, impacting aquatic environments.
6. Impact reduction :
   Transition to digital: The switch from analogue to digital radiography considerably reduces the amount of chemical waste.
   Energy savings: More efficient machines and more rational use can reduce energy consumption.
   Training and awareness: Educating staff about the importance of reducing waste and recycling can have a significant impact.

It is essential that the field of radiology takes account of its environmental impact, not only to protect the planet, but also to ensure the sustainability of its practices. Technological innovations and new approaches can help to minimise this impact while maintaining and even improving standards of care.

Green initiatives in radiology : reduce, recycle, renew

In a world that is increasingly aware of the environmental impact of its actions, radiology is no exception. Faced with today's ecological challenges, many green initiatives are emerging, seeking to align excellence in medical care with environmental responsibility. Let's see how the motto "reduce, recycle, renew" applies to this field.

1. Reduce :
   Energy consumption: With the adoption of high-efficiency equipment and intelligent energy management systems, consumption is reduced while performance is maintained.

   Radiographic waste: The switch from analogue to digital radiography eliminates the need for chemicals and reduces waste.

   Use of contrast agents: The judicious and optimised use of contrast agents minimises the quantity needed, thereby reducing waste and environmental impact.

2. Recycling :
   End-of-life equipment: Instead of sending them to landfill, obsolete machines are dismantled and their components recycled.

   Consumables: The use of recyclable materials for sheets, protective clothing and other consumables makes them easy to reuse and recycle.

   Water: Cooling systems can be designed to recycle water, minimising consumption.

3. Renew :
   Energy sources: The adoption of renewable energies, such as solar or wind power, to power radiology facilities is a growing initiative.

- **Ongoing training:** Regular training of staff in green best practice ensures that green initiatives are implemented and maintained.
- **Collaboration:** By working with suppliers committed to sustainable practices, radiology can encourage a greener supply chain.

4. Bonus - Raising awareness :

- **Information campaigns:** Raising awareness of green initiatives in radiology among staff, patients and the general public reinforces the commitment to a sustainable future.
- **Incentives:** Offering incentives, such as discounts for suppliers using recycled materials, can encourage greener practices.

Radiology is well placed to lead the movement towards more environmentally friendly healthcare. With the combination of technology, innovation and a commitment to sustainability, it is possible to provide high quality care while protecting our planet for future generations. The motto "reduce, recycle, renew" serves as the compass guiding this essential transition.

Case studies :
Eco-responsible radiology centres

Around the world, awareness of the ecological emergency is prompting more and more medical institutions to rethink the way they operate. In the field of radiology, avant-garde centres have adopted eco-responsible approaches, combining high-quality medical care with respect for the environment. Here are a few case studies illustrating these exemplary initiatives.

1. Nordica Radiological Centre (CRN), Sweden :
   - **Eco-designed building:** CRN has been designed with bioclimatic architecture, maximising the use of natural light and minimising heat loss.
   - **Innovative cooling system:** The machines are cooled using local glacial water, reducing energy consumption.
   - **Film recycling:** CRN has set up a programme to recycle X-ray film, considerably reducing waste.

2. GreenTech Imaging Center (GTEC), California, USA:
   - **Solar energy:** With a large installation of solar panels, the CIGT covers a significant part of its energy needs thanks to the sun.
   - **Zero waste programme:** everything from paper cups to medical sheets is recycled or composted, drastically reducing the amount of waste sent to landfill.
   - **Eco-responsible partnerships:** CIGT works exclusively with suppliers who share its environmental ethic.

3. Radiology Alpine EcoCentric (RAE), Switzerland :
   - **Thermal insulation:** Located in the mountains, the RAE uses local sheep's wool as insulation, offering excellent thermal performance while supporting the local economy.
   - **Eco-friendly transport:** The centre offers discounts to patients who use eco-friendly means of transport (bicycle, carpooling) to get to appointments.
   - **Raising awareness:** Workshops on eco-responsibility are regularly offered to patients and staff.

4. Centre for Bio-light Imaging (CIB), New Zealand :
   - **Water management:** The CIB uses a rainwater recovery system for non-medical needs and a water recycling system for equipment.

Therapeutic garden: An outdoor area has been designed not only for the well-being of patients, but also as an ecosystem to encourage local biodiversity.

Responsible purchasing: The centre favours the purchase of second-hand or reconditioned equipment, thereby extending the life of machines and reducing waste.

These case studies show that, whatever the size or location of a radiology centre, concrete actions can be taken to reduce its ecological footprint. Although these initiatives require an initial investment, in the long term they can offer substantial savings and position centres as leaders in the field of eco-responsibility in healthcare.

Chapter 10:
POSITIONING TECHNIQUES AND IMMOBILISATION

The art of positioning : get the best image

In radiology, a picture is worth a thousand words. The clarity, precision and quality of an X-ray image can mean the difference between a rapid, accurate diagnosis and hours of uncertainty. At the heart of this quest for excellence lies the art of positioning. Just as a photographer painstakingly adjusts his subject in the perfect light, the radiology nurse manipulates and positions the patient to get the best possible shot. Let's decipher this delicate dance between technology, anatomy and compassion.

1. Understanding anatomy :
The basis of all good positioning is a thorough understanding of human anatomy. Knowledge of bone, muscle and organ structures helps the nurse to align the patient and the equipment correctly.

   Bones and joints: The positioning of bony structures, particularly joints, is crucial for obtaining clear images.

   Organs and tissues: Depending on the type of examination, the positioning may require certain organs or tissues to be highlighted or concealed.

2. Use equipment wisely :
Control of the radiology equipment is just as essential.

   Detector plate and X-ray tube: Correct alignment between these two elements ensures a sharp, well-focused image.

Accessories: wedges, cushions and other immobilisation devices can be used to hold the patient in a specific position.

3. Communication with the patient :

Positioning can sometimes be uncomfortable. Good communication is therefore essential to put the patient at ease.

Clear instructions: Patients are not always familiar with technical terms, so it's important to give them simple, clear instructions.

Empathy: Nurses must always show empathy and patience, particularly with anxious or painful patients.

4. Specific techniques according to the examination :

Each type of radiological examination has its own positioning requirements.

Chest X-ray: For example, the patient should generally be standing with hands on hips and shoulders forward.

Radiography of the hip: The patient may be lying down with the leg turned inwards.

5. Repeat if necessary:

Even with the best positioning, it is sometimes necessary to take another shot. That's why immediate verification of image quality is crucial.

6. Keeping abreast of the latest techniques :

The art of positioning evolves with technology and research. Nurses therefore need to keep abreast of the latest techniques to provide the best possible care.

The art of positioning in radiology is an essential skill that combines science, technique and compassion. When mastered, it not only results in superior images, but also ensures an optimal patient experience. In the dance between man and machine, the radiology nurse plays the role of conductor, directing every movement to create perfect harmony.

Immobilisation techniques and equipment

In the world of radiology, movement is the enemy of a clear image. Patients can sometimes find it difficult to remain still, whether due to pain, anxiety or simply a lack of understanding of the importance of remaining static. To obtain accurate imaging, it is often necessary to use immobilisation techniques and equipment. Let's take a closer look at how this is done.

1. Why is immobilisation necessary?
- **Artefact prevention:** Any movement during shooting can create artefacts, making the image blurred or difficult to interpret.
- **Safety:** Some examinations require the patient to remain in a precise position to avoid any risk.
- **Optimising imaging:** Good, stable positioning ensures the best possible image quality.

2. Manual techniques :
Before using equipment, nurses can use manual techniques.
- **Verbal guidance:** Clear communication with the patient can often be enough to achieve the necessary immobility.
- **Physical support:** In some cases, gentle manual pressure or the placement of the nurse's hands can help stabilise an area.

3. Common immobilisers :
- **Cushions and wedges:** These moulded devices support and immobilise certain parts of the body.
- **Straps:** Straps can be used to hold limbs in place, especially for children.
- **Cervical collars:** Used to stabilise the cervical spine in cases of suspected injury.

Restraint systems for children: Devices specifically designed to gently immobilise children who may have difficulty remaining still.

4. Immobilisation for specific examinations :

Head X-ray: Special devices called head crutches can be used to stabilise the head.

Imaging the spine: Specific devices are often needed to hold the spine in place and prevent movement.

5. Special considerations :

Anxious patients: The use of relaxation techniques or the presence of someone close to you can help.

Patients with specific medical conditions: Some patients, such as those with neurodegenerative diseases, may require tailored immobilisation approaches.

6. Training and updates :

Immobilisation technology and techniques are evolving. Nurses need to be trained in the latest methods and devices available to ensure safe and effective immobilisation.

Immobilisation in radiology is both an art and a science. While technology plays a crucial role in obtaining clear images, it is the nurse's human touch, empathy and expertise that ensure that every patient is treated with care and respect. These techniques and equipment guarantee not only the quality of the images, but also the well-being and safety of the patient.

Special cases : elderly, disabled or with other specific needs

Radiology, in all its technicality, is above all a human affair. Every patient who walks through the door of the medical imaging department brings with him or her a unique set of needs, expectations and challenges. Radiology nurses are often faced with special cases, where a personalised approach is essential. Let's explore these delicate situations and the best practices for dealing with them.

1. Elderly patients :
The ageing population presents its own challenges in terms of medical imaging.

- **Reduced mobility:** Aids such as wheelchairs or walkers may be needed to move the patient.
- **Dementia or confusion:** Calm communication, reassuring gestures and sometimes the presence of a relative can help.
- **Increased sensitivity:** Older people may be more sensitive to pain or discomfort, requiring additional cushions or support.

2. Disabled patients :
Whether the disability is physical or mental, each case requires special attention.

- **Physical disability:** Adapted equipment, such as adjustable X-ray tables, may be required. Communication is key to determining the patient's specific needs.
- **Mental disability:** The approach must be patient and empathetic, with clear instructions. In some cases, light sedation may be considered.

3. Patients with specific psychological needs :
Some patients may have severe anxiety, phobia or other psychological needs.

- **Relaxation techniques:** Methods such as deep breathing or distraction can help.
- **The presence of a loved one:** Having a family member or friend close by can offer extra comfort.
- **Adapted environment:** In some centres, themed or soothing imaging rooms are available to create a less clinical environment.

4. Patients with implanted medical devices :

Pacemakers, insulin pumps, cochlear implants... all require specific preparation and precautions during imaging.

- **Preliminary check:** Before any examination, it is crucial to check for the presence of any implanted medical device.
- **Adjustable settings:** Some imaging equipment may require adjustments to avoid interfering with these devices.

The key to successful management of special cases in radiology is flexibility, communication and empathy. Radiology nurses must be trained not only in the technical aspects of their role, but also in the crucial importance of humanity in care. Ultimately, every patient is unique, and it is this individuality that makes the radiology nursing profession so valuable and rewarding.

Chapter 11:
THE CHALLENGES OF RADIOLOGY IN THE DIGITAL AGE

Teleradiology :
benefits, challenges and ethical implications

Teleradiology, which refers to the electronic transmission of radiological images from one location to another for consultation and interpretation, represents a major development in the field of radiology. It enables healthcare professionals to overcome geographical constraints, improve access to care and respond more quickly to patients' needs. However, it also presents unique challenges and ethical implications. Let's take a closer look.

1. Advantages of teleradiology :
  - **Wider access:** Hospitals and clinics in remote or underserved areas can benefit from the expertise of radiologists in major centres.
  - **24/7 availability:** Teleradiology ensures constant radiology coverage, particularly during non-working hours.
  - **Reduced turnaround times:** Results can be delivered quickly, improving patient turnaround times.
  - **Specialisation:** Teleradiology provides access to sub-specialists for complex cases.
2. The challenges of teleradiology :
  - **Technological issues:** The need for a solid infrastructure, adequate bandwidth and robust security systems.

Image quality: Ensure that the quality of the image transmitted is optimal for accurate interpretation.

Communication: Maintaining effective communication between radiologists, radiology technicians and other healthcare professionals can be more difficult at a distance.

3. Ethical implications :

Confidentiality and data security : The protection of patient data is paramount. Teleradiology systems must be secure to prevent any risk of data breach.

Quality of care: Standards of care must be maintained, regardless of where the interpretation takes place. It is essential to ensure that teleradiology does not compromise the quality of the assessment.

Responsibility: Clarifying responsibilities between the on-site radiologist and the remote radiologist is crucial.

Patient relations: In a teleradiology context, it can be more difficult to establish a direct relationship with the patient, which can influence the perception of care.

Teleradiology, while a promising technological advance, must be approached with caution and diligence. It offers the possibility of extending access to care and providing specialist expertise where it might otherwise be limited. However, it also requires increased attention to technical detail, quality of care and ethics. For radiology nurses and other professionals, this means remaining informed, adaptive and always patient-centred, even at a distance.

Data security and confidentiality in the digital age

In the digital age, data security and confidentiality have become major concerns for many sectors, and medicine is no exception. With the rapid evolution of technology, healthcare systems have adopted electronic medical records, telemedicine platforms and other digital tools to improve the efficiency of care. While these tools offer many benefits, they also present challenges when it comes to protecting sensitive patient information. Let's take a closer look at the implications of this digital transformation.

1. The rise of digital medicine :
   - **Electronic medical records:** centralising information for better monitoring and faster decision-making.
   - **Telemedicine:** Allowing remote consultations, thereby optimising access to care.
   - **Connected medical devices:** offering real-time monitoring and automated alerts for patients and healthcare professionals.
2. Advantages of digitisation :
   - **Efficiency:** Reduced waiting time, instant access to information.
   - **Accessibility:** Making it easier for different healthcare professionals to consult files.
   - **Interoperability:** Possibility of integrating various systems for a holistic view of the patient.
3. Digital risks :
   - **Attacks and breaches:** Cybercriminals may target healthcare systems to gain access to sensitive data or demand ransoms.
   - **Human error:** Data entry errors or mishandling can compromise data integrity.
   - **Technical faults:** Hardware or software faults may render data inaccessible.
4. Protecting confidentiality in the digital age :
   - **Robust security protocols :** Systems must be equipped with firewalls, anti-virus and other security measures.
   - **Staff training:** Ensuring that every member of staff is aware of the risks and knows how to protect data.

Regular updates: Software must be regularly updated to correct vulnerabilities.

Audits and assessments : Systems should be regularly assessed to identify and correct potential flaws.

5. Ethical considerations :

Informed consent: Patients must be informed and give their consent to the collection, storage and sharing of their data.

Transparency: Patients should have access to their information and know how it is used.

Responsibility: In the event of a breach, organisations must take responsibility for informing the parties concerned and taking corrective action.

While the digital age is bringing significant improvements to the delivery of medical care, it comes with its own set of challenges in terms of security and confidentiality. It is imperative that healthcare professionals, particularly those working in radiology, are well equipped and trained to navigate this complex landscape. The key is to strike a balance between exploiting the benefits of technology and ensuring patient safety and confidentiality.

Future developments :
Artificial intelligence and automation

As technology continues to advance at breakneck speed, medicine, and radiology in particular, are on the brink of a radical transformation. Artificial intelligence (AI) and automation are at the heart of this evolution, promising to increase diagnostic accuracy, improve efficiency and push back the boundaries of what we consider possible. Let's take a look at the potential implications of these technologies for the future of radiology.

1. Artificial intelligence in radiology :
    Image analysis: AI can be trained to identify and characterise anomalies in images, sometimes with an accuracy greater than or equal to that of human radiologists.

    Image enhancement: The use of algorithms to improve image quality, reduce noise and optimise imaging parameters.

2. Advantages of AI :
    Efficiency: Reduction in the time needed to analyse images, enabling more patients to be treated in less time.

    Accuracy: Minimisation of human error, reducing missed or incorrect diagnoses.

    Predictability: Using data to predict future risks or disease progression.

3. AI challenges :
    Ethics: Who is responsible if a machine makes a diagnostic error? How can we ensure that AI is used ethically?

    Training: Professionals need to be trained not only to use these tools, but also to understand their limitations.

    Cost: Setting up advanced AI systems can require significant financial investment.

4. Automation in radiology :
    Workflow: Automate repetitive tasks such as image sorting, patient tracking and appointment management.

    Predictive maintenance: Using AI to anticipate equipment maintenance needs, thereby reducing downtime.

5. Human-machine interaction :
    Complementarity: AI is not there to replace radiologists, but to complement them, by providing them with tools that increase their ability to diagnose and treat.

Trust: Building a relationship of trust between healthcare professionals and automated systems is crucial to successful adoption.

The advent of artificial intelligence and automation in radiology marks the start of a new era. While these technologies offer undeniable advantages in terms of efficiency and accuracy, they also raise ethical and practical questions that need to be approached with caution. The ultimate goal is to harmonise human expertise with the power of the machine, creating a future where technology and humanity work together to deliver healthcare of the highest quality.

Chapter 12:
PATIENT MANAGEMENT
WITH SPECIAL NEEDS

Patients with cognitive or physical disabilities

Medical imaging is a crucial stage in the care of many patients, but it can present particular challenges for those with cognitive or physical impairments. These patients have specific needs that require tailored attention and management to ensure not only the quality of care, but also their safety and comfort during X-ray examinations.

1. Understanding the patient :
    - **Demystifying disabilities:** Raising awareness of the different types of disability, whether cognitive (such as dementia, autism, mental retardation) or physical (such as paralysis, amputations).
    - **Communication:** Adopting communication techniques adapted to each patient, in particular by using visual aids or gestures.
2. Adapting the environment :
    - **Layout:** Ensure easy access to equipment, particularly for patients in wheelchairs.
    - **Comfort:** Create a soothing environment, for example by using subdued lighting or soft music for anxious or agitated patients.
3. Specific imaging techniques :
    - **Positioning:** Use specific positioning aids and techniques to ensure image clarity while guaranteeing patient comfort.

Examination duration: Anticipate the possibility that certain examinations may take longer because of the patient's particular needs.

4. Safety first:

Immobility: For patients who find it difficult to remain still, consider the use of gentle immobilisation equipment or distraction techniques.

Monitoring: Constant monitoring is essential, especially if the patient is likely to remove medical devices or move around during the examination.

5. The role of the carer :

Presence: In many cases, the presence of a familiar carer can be beneficial in reassuring and guiding the patient.

Training: Carers can be trained in simple techniques to help position and reassure the patient.

6. After the examination :

Debriefing: Take the time to explain the results of the examination to the patient and carer, using simple, understandable language.

Feedback: Soliciting feedback from patients and carers to continually improve care.

Managing patients with cognitive or physical impairments in radiology requires a holistic, patient-centred approach. By understanding their needs and adapting the environment and techniques used, it is possible to ensure a positive patient experience while obtaining the necessary diagnostic images.

Radiology at the end of life and palliative care

Radiology plays an essential role even in the final stages of a patient's life. For those in palliative care, imaging examinations can help manage pain, assess disease progression or simply improve remaining quality of life. However, the decision to use radiology in this context must be taken with discernment, balancing the potential benefits against patient comfort.

1. The importance of communication :
    Dialogue with the healthcare team: Close collaboration between radiologists, oncologists, specialist nurses and other healthcare professionals is essential to determine the best imaging strategy.
    Talking to the patient and family: Understanding the patient's wishes, clearly explaining the advantages and disadvantages of each examination, and respecting their decisions.
2. Choice of radiological examination :
    Relevance: Not all examinations are necessary. Imaging requests should be aimed at improving patient comfort or answering a specific medical question.
    Minimise discomfort: Opt for non-invasive or less uncomfortable methods whenever possible.
3. Pain and comfort management :
    Positioning: Cushions, positioning aids and other devices can be used to make the process as comfortable as possible.
    Duration: If an exam is going to be long, breaks may be necessary, or it may be useful to split the exam into several short sessions.
4. Objectives of imaging examinations :
    Pain management: Locating the cause of pain to treat it more effectively.
    Assessing progression: Although palliative care is not about cure, it is sometimes useful to know how an illness is progressing in order to adjust treatments.
    Treatment planning: Helping clinicians plan interventions to improve comfort, such as draining an effusion.

5. Ethical aspects :
- **Informed consent: Make sure** the patient and/or family understand the purpose of the examination, its risks and benefits.
- **Respecting patients' wishes:** Some patients may refuse additional tests, and these decisions must be respected.

6. Review of the exam :
- **Communication of results:** Results should be communicated quickly and in an empathetic manner, taking into account the emotional state of the patient and their family.
- **Psychological support:** Following the results, support sessions or referrals to counsellors may be necessary.

Radiology at the end of life and in a palliative care context is a challenge that requires a combination of medical, ethical and human skills. While the main objective is to improve the patient's quality of life, respect, compassion and open communication are essential to navigating this delicate area of medicine.

Appropriate communication and patient-centred approach

In radiology, as in other medical fields, communication is an essential element in ensuring effective and empathetic patient care. Every patient is unique, with his or her own concerns, medical history, needs and wishes. Adopting appropriate communication and a patient-centred approach is therefore vital to ensuring a positive experience and quality care.

1. Listen before you speak :
   - **The importance of active listening:** understanding the patient's concerns, needs and expectations by listening carefully.
   - **Open questions:** Encourage patients to share their thoughts and feelings by asking open-ended questions.
2. Adapting language :
   - **Simplicity:** Avoid medical jargon and explain technical terms in a simple, understandable way.
   - **Clarification:** Ensure that the patient has understood the information provided by asking them to rephrase it or express any questions they may have.
3. Understanding the person behind the patient :
   - **Medical history:** understanding the medical context to adapt care.
   - **Emotional state:** Recognising anxiety, fear or other emotions and offering appropriate support.
4. Non-verbal communication :
   - **Body language:** being aware of your own gestures and postures, as well as those of the patient.
   - **Eye contact:** Maintaining appropriate eye contact to show attention and presence.
5. Putting the patient at the centre of decision-making :
   - **Informed consent:** Providing all the information necessary to enable the patient to make an informed decision.
   - **Active participation:** Encourage patients to take an active part in their care, by asking questions and expressing their preferences.
6. Culture and diversity :
   - **Cultural awareness:** Respecting and understanding different cultural beliefs, values and practices.
   - **Interpreters:** Use interpreters when necessary to overcome language barriers.

7. Handling difficult situations :

   Bad news: Adopt an empathetic and transparent approach when communicating unpleasant news.

   Resistance or refusal: Understand the reasons behind the patient's negative reactions and offer alternatives or further explanations.

8. Using technology wisely :

   Telemedicine: offering remote consultations while maintaining a high level of communication and empathy.

   Electronic documentation: Ensure that data entry does not interfere with face-to-face communication.

Effective communication and a patient-centred approach in radiology involve more than simply passing on information. It's about establishing a relationship of trust, respecting patients' dignity and recognising their rights as individuals. By putting the patient at the heart of the care process, healthcare professionals can offer optimal care while enhancing patient satisfaction and well-being.

Chapter 13:
ADAPTING TO NIGHTLIFE: ROTATIONAL WORK AND EMERGENCY RADIOLOGY

Challenges and benefits shift work

Shift work is common in many sectors, particularly in the medical field, where patient care must be provided 24 hours a day, 7 days a week. This type of working schedule presents specific advantages and challenges, both for healthcare professionals and establishments. Let's look at them in a fluid and detailed way.

The challenges of working shifts :

- **Circadian rhythm disturbances:** Our bodies are set to a natural 24-hour rhythm, and any shift in this rhythm can disrupt sleep, mood and general well-being.
- **Impact on health:** Night work can increase the risk of chronic diseases such as cardiovascular disease, diabetes and obesity.
- **Fatigue and drowsiness:** Working unusual hours can lead to increased fatigue, which can potentially reduce alertness and the ability to make quick decisions.
- **Social and family life:** Irregular working hours can make it difficult to plan social or family activities, leading to feelings of isolation.
- **Occupational risks:** Working at night or early in the morning can be associated with a reduction in available resources, which can increase stress and the risk of errors.

Advantages of working shifts :

- **Night and weekend bonuses:** Many establishments offer financial compensation for hours worked during shifts.
- **Flexibility:** Some professionals appreciate being able to manage their free time during the week, avoiding the crowds and freeing up time for personal commitments.
- **Less traffic: Getting to** work at unconventional times often means avoiding traffic jams.
- **Team cohesion:** Night and weekend teams often develop a strong sense of cohesion due to the unique nature of their work.
- **Professional opportunities:** Working shifts can offer more opportunities for learning and professional growth, as you may have to take on more responsibility in the absence of administrative staff.

While working shifts presents undeniable challenges, it also offers benefits that can be very attractive to some professionals. A key to success in this way of working is to understand and manage the potential impact on health and well-being, while exploiting the positive aspects for both career and personal life. Open communication with colleagues, management and family is also essential to successfully navigate this unique professional landscape.

Tips for managing your circadian rhythm

When we work shifts, as is often the case in radiology and other medical sectors, our circadian rhythm - the internal biological clock that regulates many of our body's functions - can be disrupted. Proper management of circadian rhythm is therefore essential for maintaining good health, maximum alertness and optimum quality of life.

Here are a few tips on how to best manage your circadian rhythm when working shifts:

Create an ideal sleeping environment:

Darken your bedroom: Use opaque curtains to block out the daylight.

Minimise noise: Consider using earplugs or a white noise machine to mask outside noise.

Keep the room cool: A slightly cooler temperature helps you sleep better.

Stay regular: Even if you work shifts, try as far as possible to go to bed and get up at the same time every day.

Light exposure :

Before your night shift: Try to expose yourself to bright light, which can help signal your body that it's time to wake up.

After your night shift: Reduce your exposure to bright light, especially blue light from screens, to signal to your body that it's time to rest.

Suitable food :

Eat light at night: Avoid heavy or caffeine-rich meals during your shift.

Stay hydrated: Drinking enough water can help you stay alert.

Take active breaks: If you feel drowsy during your shift, take a moment to stretch, go for a short walk or practice deep breathing.

Limit caffeine: If you need to consume caffeine to stay awake, try to limit it at the beginning of your shift to avoid affecting your sleep afterwards.

Strategic nap: A short nap before starting your shift can help improve alertness. However, limit the nap to 20-30 minutes to avoid drowsiness.

- **Consult a sleep specialist:** If you have persistent difficulty sleeping or staying awake during your shift, it may be worth consulting a sleep specialist.
- **Avoid changing shifts frequently:** If possible, try to keep to a regular work schedule rather than constantly changing shifts.
- **Plan your rest days:** After a series of night shifts, give yourself a rest day to allow your body to readjust to a normal schedule.

Managing your circadian rhythm while working shifts is a challenge, but with the right planning and strategies, you can minimise the negative effects on your health and well-being.

The specific nature of emergency radiology

Radiology, as a discipline, has developed extensively over the years, encompassing a diverse range of procedures and imaging. However, among the many sub-disciplines of radiology, emergency radiology occupies a unique position, being at the crossroads between cutting-edge technology and the most crucial medical situations.

- What is emergency radiology?
Emergency radiology specialises in the rapid and accurate interpretation of images for patients in emergency situations. These situations can range from sudden sports injuries to car accidents and acute medical complications.
- The importance of speed :
  - **Rapid diagnosis:** One of the main roles of emergency radiology is to provide rapid diagnoses to facilitate immediate management.

Workflow optimisation: In an emergency service, every minute counts. The ability to quickly obtain and interpret an image is crucial.

Complexity   of cases :
Emergency radiologists are often faced with more complex cases than those in other disciplines, as patients may present with multiple injuries or acute medical conditions.

Interdisciplinary collaboration :
Emergency radiology requires close collaboration with other specialists, such as emergency physicians, trauma surgeons and neurologists, to name but a few.

Cutting-edge technologies :
Emergency departments are often equipped with the most advanced imaging technologies, as accurate diagnosis is essential in these critical situations.

Specialised   training :
Many radiologists choose to undertake additional training to specialise in emergency radiology, focusing on the specific skills needed to accurately interpret images in an emergency setting.

Emotional challenges :
The emergency context can be stressful not only for patients and their families, but also for medical staff. Emergency radiologists often have to work in intense situations, while remaining calm and focused.

Constant innovation:
Research and development in the field of emergency radiology is constant. New techniques and technologies emerge regularly, offering more effective methods of diagnosing and treating patients in emergency situations.

Emergency radiology is a vital and dynamic sub-discipline of radiology, combining medical expertise, cutting-edge technology and emergency management skills. Professionals working in this field play an essential role in the care of patients at the most critical moments in their lives.

Chapter 14:
THE IMPORTANCE OF SCREENING IN RADIOLOGY

Common screening techniques: mammography, bone densitometry, etc.

Screening is an essential part of medical prevention. It is the art and science of detecting diseases or abnormalities even before symptoms appear, enabling early and often more effective intervention. In the field of radiology, a number of techniques are commonly used to screen for various conditions. Let's take a look at some of these methods and their importance.

- Mammography :
  - **Definition:** Mammography is a radiological imaging technique that uses X-rays to visualise the inside of the breasts.
  - **Indication:** It is mainly used for breast cancer screening.
  - **Advantages:** This method can detect tumours before they become palpable or other symptoms appear.
  - **Digital versus analogue mammography:** Digital mammography allows more accurate viewing and electronic manipulation of images.
- Bone densitometry :
  - **Definition:** Also known as osteodensitometry, it measures bone mineral density.
  - **Indication:** It is used to screen for osteoporosis and assess the risk of fractures.

- **Principle:** This technique uses X-rays to produce images of bones, usually the spine, hip or wrist.
- Ultrasound :
  - **Definition:** Ultrasound uses sound waves to produce images of the body's internal organs.
  - **Indications:** It is often used to screen for gynaecological, obstetric and cardiac conditions.
  - **Advantages:** Non-invasive and without ionising radiation, it is safe even during pregnancy.
- Low-dose scanner for lung cancer screening :
  - **Definition:** This is a computer tomography technique that uses a low dose of radiation to visualise the lungs.
  - **Indication:** For long-term smokers or those with a significant smoking history, this method allows early detection of lung cancer.
- Virtual colonography :
  - **Definition:** Uses computer tomography to produce detailed images of the colon.
  - **Indication:** Screening for colorectal cancer and polyps.
  - **Advantages:** Non-invasive and often used as an alternative to traditional colonoscopy.
- Whole body MRI :
  - **Definition:** Whole-body magnetic resonance imaging provides a complete view of the body without the use of X-rays.
  - **Indications:** Although controversial, some people choose this method for a comprehensive assessment, particularly if there is a family history of disease.

Radiology plays a key role in screening for many diseases, enabling early detection and better health management. It is essential for healthcare professionals and patients to understand these techniques and their importance, ensuring a proactive approach to health.

Communication and managing patient anxiety

Although essential to modern medicine, radiology can often be a source of anxiety for many patients. The unknown, the noise of the machines, the feeling of being locked in an MRI machine, or simply the anticipation of the results can cause real distress. As a radiology nurse, communication is crucial not only to the effectiveness of the procedures, but also to the patient's well-being.

- Understanding patient anxiety :
  - **Causes of anxiety:** Fears may stem from physical discomfort, the unknown, exposure to radiation, or anticipation of the results.
  - **Common symptoms:** Sweating, trembling, dizziness, nausea, or even complete panic.
- Establishing open communication :
  - **First contact:** A positive, reassuring first impression can put patients at ease.
  - **Active listening:** Showing patients that their concerns are heard and taken seriously.
  - **Use clear language:** Avoid medical jargon wherever possible and provide simple explanations of the procedure.
- Relaxation techniques :
  - **Deep breathing:** A simple but effective technique for calming the nervous system.
  - **Soothing music or sound:** Some centres offer headphones with relaxing music during procedures.

- **Visualisation:** Encourage the patient to imagine a soothing place or situation.

Anticipating the patient's needs :
- **Positioning:** Make sure the patient is as comfortable as possible before starting.
- **Reassurance about the duration:** Informing the patient about the likely duration of the procedure can help to reduce anxiety.

Managing special situations :
- **Claustrophobia:** Patients with a fear of enclosed spaces may require adjustments or even mild sedation.
- **Children:** Use techniques adapted to children, such as using toys or books to divert their attention.

Post-procedure feedback :
- **Reassure the patient:** Even if the results are not immediate, tell the patient when they can expect to hear back.
- **Giving advice after the procedure:** Some patients may experience mild side effects after procedures such as contrast-enhanced scans.

Continuing education :
- **Workshops and training: Keep up to date with** the latest communication and anxiety management techniques.
- **Patient feedback:** Encourage feedback to drive continuous improvement.

Managing patient anxiety in radiology goes far beyond simply producing an image. It is a delicate balance between technology and humanity, requiring a combination of technical and interpersonal skills. By placing the patient's well-being at the heart of their mission, radiology nurses play an essential role in the success of radiological procedures and the improvement of patient care.

The crucial role of the nurse
in patient monitoring

Every day, millions of people around the world enter radiology departments, hoping for a clear diagnosis, a cure or a better understanding of their condition. While the radiologist is the one who interprets the images, the nurse is the pillar who supports the patient throughout the process. The nurse's role in monitoring radiology patients is both delicate and essential.

Pre-procedure: Preparation and assessment

Medical assessment: medical history, allergies, current medication and any contraindications to the procedure.

Patient education: Explanation of the procedure, the risks and benefits, and answers to any questions.

Informed consent: Ensuring that the patient understands and agrees to the procedure.

Support during the procedure

Emotional support: reassuring the patient, offering a reassuring presence and establishing open communication.

Clinical monitoring: monitoring vital signs, detecting abnormalities and reacting rapidly in the event of complications.

Administration of medication : Depending on the procedure, it may be necessary to administer drugs, sedatives or contrast agents.

Post-procedure: Follow-up and care

Ongoing monitoring: Monitoring for side effects or complications following the procedure.

Post-procedure advice: Inform the patient of any restrictions, medication or care that may be required.

Coordination with the medical team: Ensuring a smooth transition to other specialities or services if necessary.

Long-term monitoring

Reminders: Follow up patients for subsequent examinations, interventions or routine checks.

Continuing education: Helping patients to understand their results and make informed decisions about their care.

Psychological support: Some results can be upsetting. The nurse often offers emotional support, referring the patient to resources or specialists if necessary.

The role of intermediary

Communication: acting as a bridge between the patient and the radiologist, translating the patient's medical terms and concerns.

Referral: guiding patients to other specialities or resources according to their needs.

Continuing training and professional development

Updating skills: The world of radiology is changing fast. Nurses need to keep up to date with best practice.

Participation in research: Some nurses participate in or conduct studies to improve patient care in radiology.

The radiology nurse is not just a technician or an assistant; she is the beating heart of a well-oiled machine dedicated to the health and well-being of patients. By combining advanced clinical skills with deep empathy, she ensures that every patient is treated with respect, care and expertise. In the hustle and bustle of the radiology department, the nurse's role in patient care is absolutely crucial.

Chapter 15:
CAREER PLANNING
AND PROFESSIONAL TRANSITIONS

Career development
in the field of radiology

Radiology is a dynamic field of medicine, combining advanced clinical skills with constantly evolving technological advances. For those just starting out in this field, the opportunities for progression and development are vast and varied.

- Career start: radiology technician
  - **Initial training:** Obtain a diploma or certification from a recognised school of radiological technology.
  - **Initial responsibilities:** Assisting radiologists, carrying out basic X-rays, familiarising yourself with the equipment and safety protocols.
- Specialisation
  - **Ultrasound, mammography, MRI, CT:** each of these imaging modalities requires specific training and offers distinct opportunities.
  - **Interventional radiology:** Combination of surgical and imaging techniques for procedures such as biopsies or catheterisation.
- Nurse specialising in radiology
  - **In-depth role:** Managing patient care, administering drugs and contrast agents, working closely with radiologists.

- Supervisor or team leader
  - **Team management:** Supervising technicians, managing schedules, providing ongoing training.
  - **Interface with other departments:** Working with surgeons, oncologists and other specialists to optimise patient care.
- Radiology manager or administrator
  - **Operational management:** managing the budget, equipment and maintenance, and ensuring the overall efficiency of the department.
  - **Relations with suppliers:** Selecting and negotiating with equipment and software suppliers.
- Trainer or teacher in radiology
  - **Schools of radiological technology:** Training the next generation of technicians and professionals.
  - **Lecturer or speaker:** Sharing expertise at conferences or specialist workshops.
- Radiology researcher
  - **Clinical research:** Exploring new techniques, improvements to existing protocols or technological innovations.
  - **Collaboration:** Working with universities, laboratories and industry to advance the field.
- Radiology consultant
  - **Consulting:** Helping hospitals, clinics and businesses optimise their radiology services.
  - **Technology assessment:** Testing and recommending new equipment or software.
- Technological and digital developments
  - **Teleradiology:** reading and interpreting images remotely.

Artificial intelligence: Working with engineers to develop tools to assist reading and interpreting.

Back to school

Pursue a specialisation or doctorate: deepen your skills or move into research.

Ongoing training: Keeping up to date with the latest developments in the field.

Career development in radiology is as diverse as it is exciting. Whether you choose to specialise in a particular modality, or move into management, teaching or research, the opportunities are immense and allow everyone to chart their own professional path.

Considerations for nurses contemplating transition to other specialities or roles

A nurse's career is often marked by a series of transitions and evolutions, driven by personal aspirations, professional opportunities, or simply the desire for change. Considering a transition to another specialty or role can be a challenging but complex decision. Here are some key considerations to help you on your way.

Self-diagnosis and introspection

Motivations: What is driving your desire for change? Are you looking for new challenges, a better quality of life, or do you have specific career aspirations?

Skills and competencies: What are your strengths and weaknesses? How do they compare with the requirements of the new role or speciality?

- Information on the new speciality/role
  - **Responsibilities and tasks:** What does this new role entail in practical terms? What will your typical day be like?
  - **Training and qualifications:** What level of training is required? Are any specific qualifications required?
- Practical considerations
  - **Impact on your personal life:** Will the new role require you to work longer or staggered hours? How will this affect your work/life balance?
  - **Financial outlook:** Are there any financial implications, whether in terms of salary, training or other associated costs?
- Training and preparation
  - **Courses and qualifications:** Find out more about the training programmes and courses available.
  - **Internships and mentoring:** An internship or mentoring in the new field can provide valuable experience and practical insights.
- Networking
  - **Talk to professionals:** Talk to people who are already working in the speciality or role you're aiming for. Their feedback can be invaluable.
  - **Attending seminars and conferences:** These events can provide learning and networking opportunities.
- Impact on long-term career
  - **Development opportunities:** How will this transition influence your career in the long term? Will it open doors to other roles or specialities?
  - **Fit with personal goals:** Is this transition in line with your long-term aspirations?

- Mental and emotional preparation
  - **Managing uncertainty:** All change involves a degree of uncertainty. Are you ready to manage the challenges and moments of discomfort that may arise?
  - **Self-confidence:** Cultivating confidence in your skills and your ability to adapt is crucial to a successful transition.
- Feedback and assessment
  - **Seeking feedback:** Once the transition has begun, seek regular feedback to help you improve.
  - **Personal assessment:** Take time to reflect on what's working and what needs adjusting.

The transition to a new specialty or a different role as a nurse is a journey that requires reflection, preparation and adaptability. Each stage, from the initial choice to integration into the new role, is an opportunity for learning and personal and professional growth.

Retirement and post-career : reflection and preparation

The prospect of retirement, after a dedicated career as a radiology nurse, often evokes a range of emotions: from excitement to nostalgia, not to mention a certain amount of apprehension. Preparing for this new stage of life requires as much care, thought and preparation as starting or mid-career. Here's a guide to tackling this transition in an informed and serene way.

- Awareness and anticipation
  - **Thinking about retirement:** What does retirement mean to you? Is it a time to rest, a

time to pursue other passions, or a combination of both?

- **Financial planning:** Assess your savings, investments and medical cover. Consult a financial advisor to plan optimally.

Health and well-being

- **Medical assessment:** Carry out a full health check to identify and prevent any health problems.
- **Physical activity and nutrition:** Adopt a healthy lifestyle to make the most of this new stage.

New horizons and passions

- **Leisure and hobbies: This is** the time to explore activities that time or professional responsibilities didn't allow before.
- **Community involvement:** Think about giving back, whether through volunteering or other forms of involvement.

Emotion and psychological support

- **Managing emotions:** Retirement is a significant step that can give rise to melancholy or anxiety. Consider seeking professional help to manage these emotions.
- **Networking with retirees:** Talk to colleagues who are already retired to get advice and share experiences.

Continuing education and training

- **Courses and workshops:** Retirement offers an opportunity to learn and develop new skills, whether for pleasure or for professional retraining.

Travel and exploration

- **Discover the world:** If conditions allow, consider travelling to discover new cultures and landscapes.

- **Educational trips :** Take part in organised trips on specific themes to combine fun and learning.

Back to the profession

- **Mentoring and coaching:** Use your experience to guide and advise young professionals.
- **Part-time consultancy:** If you're not ready to leave the professional world altogether, consider part-time consultancy or teaching roles.

Taking stock and sharing experience

- **Writing or blogging:** Consider sharing your experience and thoughts through writing, whether in a book, a blog or articles.

Retirement is a time of rebirth, exploration and self-discovery. With careful preparation, it can be one of life's most rewarding and satisfying periods.

Chapter 16:
RADIATION DOSE MANAGEMENT:
SAFETY AND EDUCATION

Importance of dose minimisation

Radiology is a fascinating and essential part of modern medicine, but it comes with its own challenges, particularly when it comes to radiation exposure. Although technological advances have considerably reduced the risks associated with medical imaging, the importance of minimising the radiation dose received by the patient remains paramount. Here's why.

- Reducing risks for the patient :
    - **Stochastic effects:** Radiation can increase the risk of developing cancer. Although the risk associated with a single examination is low, it is not zero.
    - **Deterministic effects:** High doses can cause direct tissue damage, such as burns or ulcers.
- Protection of medical staff :
    - Staff who regularly work with radiological equipment are also exposed to radiation. Minimising the dose is essential to protect their long-term health.
- Good medical practice :
    - The ALARA principle ("As Low As Reasonably Achievable") is widely adopted in radiology. It insists that any exposure to radiation must be justified and as low as reasonably achievable.
    - Justification of a procedure implies that the benefits for the patient outweigh the potential risks.

Children and sensitive populations:
> Children are more sensitive to radiation than adults. Their cells divide rapidly, making them more vulnerable. What's more, they have a longer life ahead of them, which increases the risk of developing cancer following exposure to radiation.

> Certain groups, such as pregnant women, also require special attention in terms of radiation protection.

Diagnostic effectiveness :
> Minimising the dose does not mean compromising image quality. Thanks to modern technologies, it is possible to obtain high quality images with reduced doses.

Patient confidence :
> Informing patients about the measures taken to minimise their exposure increases their confidence in the care they receive.

Ethical and legal responsibility :
> Healthcare professionals have an ethical obligation to do no harm ("primum non nocere"). They are also required by law to comply with radiation protection standards.

Dose minimisation is at the heart of modern radiology. It reflects an ongoing commitment to patient safety, quality of care and professional excellence. As technology continues to advance, it is imperative that professionals remain vigilant and informed to ensure the well-being of all those involved.

Radiation protection techniques for patients and professionals

Radiation protection is an essential component of radiological practice. It aims to protect both patients and healthcare professionals from the potentially harmful effects of ionising radiation. In a field where exposure to radiation is a daily necessity, adopting effective radiation protection techniques is not only an ethical responsibility, but also a legal obligation.

1. For the patient :

- **Justification of the examination:** Before carrying out a radiological examination, it is essential to ensure that it is medically justified. This involves weighing up the potential benefits against the risks associated with exposure to radiation.
- **Dose optimisation:** Use the lowest possible setting to obtain a quality diagnostic image. Modern machines have parameters that automatically adapt the dose according to age, size and anatomical region.
- **Lead protection:** Use lead shields, aprons and collars to protect sensitive areas that do not need to be irradiated.
- **Avoiding unnecessary X-rays:** Do not repeat X-rays unless absolutely necessary.
- **Communication:** Informing patients of the risks and benefits, and obtaining their informed consent.

2. For professionals :

- **Distance :** The amount of radiation received is inversely proportional to the square of the distance. In other words, the further away you are from the source, the less radiation you receive.
- **Shielding:** Use lead screens or booths to protect yourself during exposure.

- **Exposure time:** Minimise the time spent near the radiation source. Every second counts.
- **Personal protection:** Always wear a lead apron, protective goggles and other personal protective equipment when working near sources of radiation.
- **Monitoring:** Wear personal dosimeters to monitor and record your cumulative exposure.
- **Training:** Make sure you are regularly trained and informed about best practice in radiation protection.
- **Equipment maintenance:** Ensuring that all equipment is regularly checked and maintained to ensure that it is operating optimally and safely.
- **Work protocols:** Have clear protocols on how to carry out examinations, so as to limit radiation exposure as much as possible.

Radiation protection is an ongoing commitment to ensuring patient and professional safety. It requires constant awareness, ongoing training, and regular updating of knowledge and skills. Ultimately, it represents a balance between ensuring quality patient care while minimising the risks associated with radiation exposure.

Educating patients about risks and benefits of delisting

It is common for patients to be anxious about undergoing examinations that use radiation, mainly because of concerns about health risks. As a healthcare professional, it is your responsibility to inform and educate patients, offering clear explanations and answering any questions they may have. This can help to reduce the patient's anxiety and obtain their cooperation during the examination.

1. Introduction to radiation
    Definition: Simply explain what radiation is and how it interacts with the body.
    Types of radiation: Distinguish between ionising radiation (such as X-rays) and non-ionising radiation (such as ultrasound).
2. Advantages of radiation in medicine
    Accurate diagnosis: Radiation provides detailed images of the inside of the body, making it easier to detect a wide range of pathologies.
    Therapeutic interventions: In certain situations, such as radiotherapy, radiation is used to treat diseases.
    Less invasive: Many radiological examinations avoid the need for more invasive procedures.
3. Risks associated with radiation
    Accumulated exposure: Discuss how exposure to radiation accumulates over time.
    Probability of cell damage: Although low, there is a risk of ionising radiation damaging the DNA of cells.
    Risks for specific populations: Pregnant women and children are more sensitive to the effects of radiation.
4. Safety and prevention measures
    Minimisation of dose: Underline the commitment of medical staff to use the minimum dose required.
    Protective equipment: Explain the use of shields, lead aprons and other equipment to protect certain parts of the body.
    Regular checks on equipment: Assure the patient that the equipment is regularly checked to ensure its safety and effectiveness.
5. Importance of informed consent
    Full information: Ensuring that the patient understands the benefits and risks associated with the procedure.

Freedom of choice: Patients must feel free to ask questions, express concerns and make an informed decision.

6. Addressing concerns and myths

Clarification: Correct any misconceptions the patient may have about radiation.

Credible references: Direct patients to reliable resources if they wish to learn more.

Educating the patient is a crucial step in ensuring understanding and cooperation. A well-informed patient is more likely to follow instructions, which can lead to more effective diagnostic or therapeutic results. By taking the time to explain and reassure, you reinforce the patient's confidence in the care provided.

Chapter 17:
PATIENT CARE WITH SPECIAL NEEDS

Radiology and patients
with autism spectrum disorders

The management of patients with autism spectrum disorders (ASD) in radiology presents unique challenges for healthcare professionals. These patients may have specific needs and varied reactions to the radiological environment, requiring a personalised approach. However, with adequate preparation and a thorough understanding of the particularities of these patients, it is possible to provide them with an optimal experience.

1. Understanding the autism spectrum
   Definition and variability: It is essential to recognise that autism is a spectrum, with a wide range of symptoms and levels of functioning.
   Sensory sensitivities: Many individuals with ASD may be hypersensitive or hyposensitive to certain stimuli, such as bright lights or loud noises.
2. Upstream preparation
   Liaison with carers: Discuss with parents or carers to obtain information about the patient's idiosyncrasies, preferences and potential triggers.
   Pre-examination visits: If possible, allow the patient to visit the radiology department before the examination to familiarise themselves with the environment.
   Visual resources: Use sequences of images or videos to show the patient what to expect during the examination.

3. Adapting the environment

   Stimulus reduction: Reduce bright lights and loud noises, which can be disturbing for the patient.

   Secure areas: Provide a quiet, secure area where patients can relax before the examination.

   Distraction tools: Suggest familiar objects or sensory toys to help the patient relax.

4. Appropriate communication

   Clear, concrete language: Use simple sentences and avoid figurative expressions.

   Visual aids: Supplement verbal explanations with visual aids, such as drawings or pictograms.

   Check understanding: Make sure the patient has understood the instructions and expectations.

5. Flexibility during the exam

   Allocate more time: Recognise that some patients with ASD may need more time to feel comfortable and co-operate.

   Presence of a carer: If it helps the patient to relax, allow a relative or carer to stay close by during the examination.

6. After the examination

   Positive feedback: Praise the patient for his or her cooperation, whatever the challenges encountered.

   Suggestions for future visits: Ask carers for feedback on what worked and what could be improved for future visits.

Caring for patients with ASD in radiology requires empathy, patience and adaptability. By being committed to providing a positive experience and understanding the unique needs of these patients, radiology professionals can ensure the highest quality of care for all.

Adapting the procedure for patients suffering from anxiety disorders

Despite its undeniable diagnostic benefits, radiology can be a source of anxiety for many patients. For those who already have anxiety disorders, the experience can be particularly distressing. As a healthcare professional, adapting your approach to these patients is not only a question of caring, but also of medical effectiveness. Here are some steps and recommendations to help you better support these patients:

1. Early identification and communication
    Medical history: Check whether the patient has a history of anxiety disorders when taking medical information.
    Open dialogue: Encourage patients to express any fears or concerns they may have about the procedure.
2. Upstream preparation
    Pre-visits: Allowing patients to visit the radiology department in advance to familiarise themselves with the environment.
    Educational resources: Provide brochures, videos or other information materials that describe the procedure in detail.
3. Adapting the environment
    Soothing atmosphere: Use subdued lighting and soft colours, and consider playing soft music if it suits the patient.
    Emotional support: If it helps the patient to relax, allow them to have a relative or therapist by their side.
4. Relaxation techniques
    Guided breathing: Encourage the patient to adopt deep breathing techniques to relax.

- **Distraction:** Offer headphones to listen to music or a podcast during the procedure, if feasible.
5. Reassuring presence of staff
    - **Empathy:** Show understanding, listen actively and reassure the patient of the team's professionalism.
    - **Clear communication:** Inform the patient step by step of what is happening, avoid surprises.
6. Possibility of medication
    - **Mild sedatives:** In cases of very high anxiety, discuss the possibility of administering a mild sedative after consultation with the treating doctor.
7. After the examination
    - **Debriefing:** Take a moment to discuss the experience with the patient, so that they can express their feelings.
    - **Feedback for improvement:** Ask the patient if they have any suggestions for making the experience less anxiety-provoking in the future.

Managing patients with anxiety disorders in radiology requires increased sensitivity to the patient's emotional and psychological needs. By recognising and actively addressing these needs, professionals can not only improve the patient experience, but also achieve better diagnostic results through patient cooperation.

Techniques for managing claustrophobic patients

Claustrophobia is an intense fear of confined spaces. In radiology, this can pose particular problems during examinations such as MRI, where the patient lies in a narrow machine. Understanding and managing this fear is essential to ensuring a positive experience for the patient and obtaining quality images. Here are some techniques for dealing with claustrophobia in radiology:

1. Preliminary assessment

Questionnaire: Include questions about claustrophobia when taking the patient's history. This helps to detect any apprehensions beforehand.

2. Preparation and information

Detailed explanation: Describe the procedure in detail, explaining how long the examination will take, any noises the patient may hear, etc.

Tour of the department: If possible, give the patient a tour of the MRI room before the examination so that they can familiarise themselves with the machine and the environment.

3. Adapting the environment

Mirrors: Some MRI equipment is fitted with mirrors that allow the patient to see outside the tube, giving a feeling of space.

Light: Soft lighting or colour-changing light inside the tube may help to relax some patients.

4. Communication during the examination

Constant contact: Make sure the patient knows they can contact the technician at any time. Provide a means, such as a bell or balloon, to signal if they need a break.

Regular update: Inform the patient regularly of the time remaining for the examination.

5. Relaxation techniques

Breathing: Encourage the patient to practise deep breathing to reduce anxiety.

Music or guided meditation: Using headphones to listen to soft music or guided meditation can help to distract and calm the patient.

6. Use of sedatives

If relaxation techniques are not enough, discuss the possibility of administering a mild sedative with the attending physician.

7. Alternatives to traditional MRI

Open MRI: If your establishment has it, offer an examination with an open MRI, which is less confining.

8. Support

Reassuring presence: For some patients, the presence of someone close to them during the examination (as long as this does not affect the quality of the images) can help.

Dealing with claustrophobia in radiology requires patience, empathy and adaptability. By taking the time to understand the patient's needs and using appropriate techniques, it is possible to create a more comfortable experience for the patient while ensuring quality images for diagnosis.

Chapter 18:
EMERGING TECHNOLOGIES AND THE FUTURE OF RADIOLOGY

A look at potential developments medical imaging

Medical imaging has been on a remarkable journey since the discovery of X-rays in 1895. At the intersection of technology and medicine, this field has continued to evolve, improving diagnostic accuracy, patient comfort and the workflow of healthcare professionals. Let's take a look at the trends and innovations that could shape the future of medical imaging.

1. Artificial Intelligence (AI) and machine learning
   - **Analysis and interpretation:** AI could help detect subtle anomalies, often invisible to the human eye, making diagnoses more accurate.
   - **Optimisation of imaging protocols:** AI could adjust equipment parameters in real time to obtain the best possible images.
2. Hybrid imaging
   - Combining imaging modalities such as PET-MRI or PET-CT to provide complementary information, improving diagnosis and therapeutic planning.
3. 3D imaging and augmented reality
   - Surgeons could use interactive three-dimensional images to plan and simulate complex surgical procedures.
4. Radiomics :
   - Radiomics aims to extract a large number of characteristics from medical images, paving the way

for more detailed analyses of tumours and pathologies.

5. Advances in contrast
   Development of new, safer and more specific contrast agents for different pathologies.

6. Molecular imaging :
   Visualisation of biochemical processes at the molecular level, offering the potential for early detection of disease.

7. More eco-responsible equipment :
   Designing equipment that uses less radiation or harmful chemicals, in line with green initiatives.

8. Portability and teleradiology :
   With technological advances, imaging could become more mobile, enabling remote diagnosis and offering solutions for remote or under-equipped regions.

9. Radiation-free imaging :
   Research into imaging modalities that do not use radiation, such as certain forms of ultrasound or MRI.

10. Immersive training :
    Using virtual and augmented reality to train imaging professionals, immersing them in virtual scenarios for an in-depth learning experience.

The potential evolution of medical imaging promises to revolutionise the way diseases are diagnosed, treated and managed. By integrating the latest technologies and placing the patient at the heart of every innovation, the future of medical imaging looks both exciting and promising, with continuous improvements in patient care.

Impact of artificial intelligence and robotics

The arrival of artificial intelligence (AI) and robotics in the field of radiology is comparable to the emergence of X-rays at the beginning of the 20th century. These technologies are radically changing the way we perceive, analyse and use medical images. Let's take a look at their impact on the profession, patients and the quality of care.

1. Improved diagnosis :
   Early detection: AI can identify anomalies with astounding accuracy, sometimes even before they are visible to the human eye. This can enable early intervention and improve prognosis.

   Reducing errors: AI offers a second opinion, minimising interpretation errors and avoiding misdiagnoses or missed diagnoses.
2. Optimised workflow :
   Automation of routine tasks: AI can take care of repetitive tasks, such as image segmentation or annotation, freeing up staff time.

   Prioritisation of urgent cases: The AI can triage examinations according to severity, ensuring that cases requiring immediate attention are treated as a priority.
3. Robotics in interventional radiology :
   Robots can assist radiologists in invasive procedures, improving accuracy, reducing procedure times and minimising radiation for staff.
4. Personalised care :
   AI can analyse thousands of images to determine the best imaging modalities and parameters for a specific patient.
5. Enhanced radiation protection :
   Thanks to AI, it is possible to obtain high-quality images with lower radiation doses, thereby reducing the risks to patients.
6. Training and education :
   AI systems can be used as teaching tools for radiology students, providing them with real-time

feedback and helping with the continuing education of professionals.

7. Remote assistance :

The combination of teleradiology and AI enables radiologists to provide accurate diagnoses even from a distance, which is particularly useful for remote or under-equipped regions.

8. Anticipating ethical challenges :

With the increasing adoption of AI, it is essential to establish ethical guidelines to ensure patient confidentiality, transparency of decisions and absence of bias in algorithms.

While AI and robotics in radiology open up exciting prospects, it is crucial to remember that they are there to complement, not replace, the role of the radiologist. Human expertise, compassion and clinical judgement remain at the heart of the profession. However, with these tools, radiologists are better equipped to provide quality, accurate and personalised care to their patients.

Ethical considerations on future innovations

Radiology, at the crossroads of technology and medicine, is constantly evolving. Each new advance offers exciting prospects for improving diagnosis and treatment. However, these innovations are not without ethical concerns. Let's delve into these challenges and think about the best ways to navigate them.

1. Artificial Intelligence (AI): Friend or foe?

AI reliability: How can we ensure that the decisions made by AI are correct? Blind trust in technology can lead to medical errors.

Education and training: If young radiologists rely too heavily on AI, is there a risk that they will not fully develop their diagnostic skills?

2. Confidentiality in the digital age :

Data protection : With more and more patient data going online, how can we guarantee its security?

Patient consent : Are patients sufficiently informed about how their data is used, particularly in research?

3. Accessibility of new technologies :

Disparities in care: Can all healthcare establishments afford the latest innovations? Is there a risk of widening the gap between well-equipped centres and others, particularly in less developed regions?

4. Patient autonomy and the "right not to know" :

With the increasing precision of imaging techniques, we can detect abnormalities that are not relevant to the patient's current medical problem. When and how should patients be informed of these 'chance finds'?

5. Robotics and the dehumanisation of care:

If robots play an increasing role in procedures, how can the human and empathetic aspect of care be maintained? Is there a risk that the doctor-patient relationship will be altered?

6. Genetic evolution and imaging :

New imaging techniques could eventually provide information on genetic susceptibility to certain diseases. Does this raise ethical questions about confidentiality and discrimination?

7. Ethical implications of the research :

How can we ensure that clinical trials involving new imaging techniques are carried out ethically, particularly in vulnerable populations?

Innovations in radiology, although extremely beneficial, raise many ethical questions. To ensure patient-centred care, it is crucial that radiology professionals remain vigilant, keep themselves regularly informed and engage in ethical dialogue on these issues. Ethics must go hand in hand with technology, ensuring that every advance is made in the best interests of the patient.

Chapter 19:
PROFESSIONAL DEVELOPMENT

Keeping up to date:
Importance of continuing training

In the dynamic and technologically advanced medical field of radiology, the status quo is not an option. Healthcare professionals, including radiology nurses, find themselves at the cutting edge of constantly evolving discoveries, innovations and methodologies. That's why continuing education is not only desirable, it's essential. Here's an in-depth look at its importance.

1. Constantly evolving technology
One of the most striking aspects of radiology is the rapid pace of technological progress. From more precise imaging machines to sophisticated analysis software and the integration of artificial intelligence, keeping up to date is crucial. Continuing education provides professionals with the skills they need to master these tools.

2. Improving the quality of care
With greater knowledge and in-depth training, nurses can offer better quality care. Understanding the nuances of new techniques or best practices can mean the difference between an accurate diagnosis and a potential error.

3. Risk reduction
Radiology, although incredibly beneficial, involves risks, particularly in terms of exposure to radiation. Ongoing training enables professionals to understand these risks and learn the best methods for minimising them.

4. Professional development

In a competitive field, standing out is essential. Nurses who invest in their continuing education show a commitment to their profession, which can open doors to advanced opportunities or specialisations.

5. Meeting regulatory requirements

Many countries and regions have specific continuing education requirements for healthcare professionals. Keeping up to date with these requirements is essential if you are to maintain your licence or certification.

6. Commitment to the patient

Patients expect to receive the highest possible quality of care. By investing in continuing education, nurses demonstrate their commitment to providing exceptional care, thereby boosting patient confidence.

7. Adaptability to changing patient needs

As diseases and conditions evolve, so does the way we diagnose and treat them. Continuing education prepares nurses to adapt to these changes, ensuring optimal patient care.

Continuing education in radiology is not a luxury, but a necessity. It embodies the professional's commitment to excellence, to renewal and to providing the best possible care. In a world where technology and methods evolve rapidly, keeping up to date is the key to success and excellence in healthcare.

Specialisation and certification in radiology

Radiology is a broad field with a range of specialties that allow nurses and technologists to focus on specific areas.

While all radiology professionals share a core set of skills, specialisation can deepen knowledge in specific areas, improve the quality of care and open doors to advanced opportunities. Certification is often a guarantee of this expertise.

1. Why specialise?

In-depth expertise: Specialisation enables you to develop cutting-edge skills in a particular area of radiology, such as MRI, mammography or interventional radiology.

Career opportunities: Specialisation may lead to leadership roles, teaching positions or research in specific fields.

Professional satisfaction: Mastering a particular sub-field can offer deep satisfaction by contributing to the advancement of the profession.

2. Current areas of specialisation

Interventional radiology: A discipline based on the use of images to guide minimally invasive medical procedures.

Mammography: Focus on imaging the breast to detect cancer and other abnormalities.

Paediatric imaging: Radiology specifically adapted to the needs of children.

Neuroradiology: Imaging of the nervous system, including the brain, spinal cord and nerves.

Musculoskeletal radiology: Focus on bones, joints and associated soft tissues.

3. The certification process

Advanced training: Before qualifying for certification, it is often necessary to undergo additional training, whether in the form of courses, workshops or residency programmes.

Examination: Certification generally requires passing an examination specific to the area of specialisation.

Renewal: As with most professional qualifications, it may be necessary to renew certification on a regular basis, which often involves ongoing training.

4. The importance of certification

Professional recognition: Certification is a guarantee of competence in a given field and is often sought by employers.

Improved quality of care: Certification guarantees that the professional has the knowledge and skills required to provide high-quality care.

Commitment to the profession: Seeking certification demonstrates a commitment to excellence in the field of radiology.

Specialising and obtaining certification in radiology are steps that allow nurses and technologists to stand out in their field, offer exceptional care and develop professionally. In a constantly evolving medical sector, striving for excellence is always a priority.

Well-being and stress management : Taking care of yourself to take care of others

The medical field, with its demanding nature and often onerous responsibilities, can place considerable pressure on healthcare professionals. For radiology nurses, where precision, patience and compassion are essential, personal well-being is not just a luxury, but a necessity. In this chapter, we delve into the importance of taking care of ourselves in order to be able to take care of others.

1. Recognising burn-out and work-related stress

Symptoms of burn-out: Emotional exhaustion, cynicism, feelings of ineffectiveness, and physical symptoms such as fatigue, sleep disorders and headaches.

Risk factors: Long hours, lack of support, pressure for accurate diagnoses, and the constant need to empathise with patients.

2. The importance of work-life balance

Definition: Work-life balance is the ability to divide one's time and resources between professional and personal obligations.

Consequences of a lack of balance: exhaustion, strained personal relationships, reduced quality of care, and health risks.

3. Stress management strategies

Relaxation techniques: meditation, yoga, deep breathing techniques and visualisation.

Spending quality time: Valuing breaks, taking holidays, spending time with loved ones and enjoying hobbies.

Setting limits: Saying no, delegating tasks and taking regular breaks.

4. Importance of physical health

Balanced diet: Eat a variety of foods, avoid excess and stay hydrated.

Physical activity: Incorporate exercise into your routine, whether it's a brisk walk, jogging, dancing or any other activity that gets you moving.

Sleep: Valuing quality sleep, maintaining a regular sleep schedule and creating an environment conducive to rest.

5. Mental and emotional health

Social support: Share your concerns with colleagues, friends or family, and don't hesitate to seek professional help.

Hobbies and pastimes: Find activities that relax and excite, whether it's reading, art, music or cooking.

Resilience training: Developing the ability to bounce back from difficult situations, using stress management techniques and a positive outlook.

Taking care of oneself is not a selfish act, but a necessity for those on the front line of patient care. By valuing wellbeing and stress management, radiology nurses can not only improve their quality of life, but also the quality of care they provide. After all, a well-rested, balanced and happy carer is an effective carer.

Conclusion:

Final thoughts :
The impact of the radiology nurse

As you explore the many facets of the radiology nurse's role, you quickly discover that it's not just a technical profession. It's a vocation that demands both skill and compassion, precision and patience. In this concluding chapter, we seek to highlight the profound impact that these health professionals have, not just on medicine, but on the lives of every patient they encounter.

1. More than just a technique
The radiology nurse is the link between medical technology and the patient. She is not just the one who positions the patient or administers a contrast medium. She is also the one who reassures, listens and guides. Her ability to combine technical expertise with a human touch makes all the difference.

2. A lasting impact on patients
The image can diagnose, but it is the carer who heals. Patients often remember the machine less than the nurse who supported them during a procedure. That moment of compassion, that reassuring exchange, that hand held firmly can leave an indelible impression.

3. The pivotal role in a multidisciplinary team
Within a clinic or hospital, the radiology nurse is often the link between several specialists. They work with radiologists, technologists, referring physicians and other professionals to ensure comprehensive patient care. Their versatility and ability to communicate effectively are essential to the success of the treatment process.

4. The constant evolution of the profession

In the age of digital technology and artificial intelligence, the field of radiology is constantly evolving. Radiology nurses don't just acquire skills; they continue to adapt, learn and grow. Her dedication to continuing education is a testament to her commitment to professional excellence.

5. A heritage of humanity in a world of technology

Technology may evolve, but humanity's fundamental needs - to be listened to, understood, reassured - remain constant. The radiology nurse, despite technical advances, remains a poignant reminder that medicine, at its heart, is an art of humanity.

Reflecting on the impact of the radiology nurse, we are led to recognise that every gesture, every word, every action carries weight. This book has attempted to cover the depth and complexity of this profession, but in the end, the essence of the profession lies in those intangible moments of humanity. It is a call to every radiology nurse to fully embrace their role, as they shape not only the future of medicine, but also the hearts and minds of those they serve.

Additional resources : Where to find out more

To embark on the world of radiology is to embark on a journey of continuous learning. To help our readers navigate this vast ocean of information, we have compiled a list of essential resources that will provide you with additional depth and perspective on the topics covered in this book.

1. Books and specialised publications
   - **"Essentials of Radiographic Physics and Imaging"** by James Johnston and Terri L. Fauber: A comprehensive book on the basics of radiology.
   - **"Radiology Nursing: Scope and Standards of Practice"**: An essential guide for radiology nurses.
   - **"Journal of Radiology Nursing**: A specialist academic journal covering the latest research and best practice.
2. Websites and educational platforms
   - **RadiologyInfo.org**: Managed by the American College of Radiology (ACR) and the Radiological Society of North America (RSNA), this site offers a wealth of information for patients and professionals.
   - **AuntMinnie.com**: A news and continuing education portal for radiology professionals.
   - **RSNA.org**: The official website of the Radiological Society of North America offers educational resources, news and information on upcoming events.
3. Organisations and Associations
   - **American College of Radiology (ACR)**: A major organisation offering certification, training and resources for professionals.
   - **Association for Radiologic & Imaging Nursing (ARIN)**: Dedicated to radiology nurses, it offers training, certification and networking opportunities.
4. Conferences and seminars
   - **RSNA Annual Meeting**: A must-attend event for radiology professionals, it features the latest technological advances, educational sessions and networking opportunities.
   - **European Congress of Radiology (ECR)**: An event similar to the RSNA, but focused on Europe.
5. Online courses and Webinars
   - **Radiopaedia.org**: A free online radiology learning resource with courses, quizzes and articles.

Coursera & edX: These online learning platforms offer radiology-related courses designed by leading universities and institutions.

6. Podcasts and Videos

Radiology Firing Line (RFL): A podcast featuring interviews with experts and opinion leaders in the field of radiology.

Radiology Channel on YouTube: Educational videos, demonstrations and interviews to complement your learning.

In a constantly evolving field like radiology, it's crucial to stay up to date and informed. We hope that these resources will serve as a springboard for you to deepen your knowledge and enrich your career.

Acknowledgements :
The people who make our work possible

Writing this book has been no mean feat, and the road to achieving it has been paved with invaluable experiences, learning and collaborations. Beyond the pages of this book, there are a multitude of individuals whose support, perseverance and contributions have made this adventure possible. It's time to express my gratitude to all of them.

To my mentors
To the radiologists and healthcare professionals who have guided me through the intricacies of radiology and shared their clinical wisdom, a huge thank you. Your passion for the profession has inspired me every step of the way.

To all radiology nurses
Each testimonial, each story shared was a brick in the construction of this book. Your dedication to the well-being of patients is the beating heart of our profession. Your anecdotes and experiences have brought this text to life.

To the editorial team

Thank you for your infinite patience, your constructive feedback and your ability to transform my words into a fluid and accessible narrative. Without you, this book would be nothing more than a collection of scattered notes.

To the patients

For your trust and courage, for every question you ask, every smile you share, every tear you shed, I am eternally grateful. You are the daily reminder of why we do what we do.

To my family and friends

For your unwavering support, for being my lifeline during difficult times, for celebrating every little victory, I owe it all to you. Your love and encouragement have carried me through.

To you, dear readers

Finally, thank you for holding this book in your hands. Whether you are a curious novice or a veteran of the field, I hope you will find this guide useful and enrich your understanding of radiology. Your quest for knowledge is the raison d'être of this book.

Radiology, like all medical fields, is a team effort. This work is a reflection of that collaboration. To all those who have crossed my path and made this journey unforgettable, from the bottom of my heart, thank you.

Glossary of key terms

Angiography: Imaging technique that uses X-rays to visualise blood vessels.

Biometrics: Measurement of physical or biological characteristics.

CT (or CAT scan): Computed tomography, also known as CAT scan, is an imaging technique that uses X-rays to create detailed images of organs, bones and other tissues.

Densitometry: Measurement of density, often used to assess bone density.

Ultrasound: Imaging technique that uses sound waves to create images of internal organs.

Fluoroscopy: Imaging technique that uses X-rays to obtain images in real time, often used during medical procedures.

MRI: Magnetic Resonance Imaging, an imaging technique that uses magnetic fields to obtain detailed images.

Isotope: Form of an element with the same number of protons but a different number of neutrons.

Mammography: X-ray examination of the breasts, used mainly for breast cancer screening.

:PACS Picture Archiving and Communication System. This is a computer system that stores, retrieves, distributes and presents medical images.

Radiography: Imaging technique that uses X-rays to visualise the internal structures of the body.

Radiation protection: All means of protection against ionising radiation.

Scanner: See CT/CT.

Teleradiology: the practice of radiology at a distance, where images are transmitted from one place to another for interpretation and/or consultation.

Thermography: Imaging technique that detects heat to create an "image" of the temperature distribution of an area of the body.

Ultrasound: High-frequency sound waves used in ultrasound.

This glossary provides an overview of terms commonly used in radiology. For a more in-depth definition or information on specific terms not included here, it is recommended that you consult specialist resources in the field of radiology.

Scientific and medical references

Bushberg, J. T., Seibert, J. A., Leidholdt Jr, E. M., & Boone, J. M. (2011). *The Essential Physics of Medical Imaging* (3rd ed.). Lippincott Williams & Wilkins.

Cherry, S. R., Sorenson, J. A., & Phelps, M. E. (2012). *Physics in Nuclear Medicine* (4th ed.). Elsevier.

Hendee, W. R., & Ritenour, E. R. (2002). *Medical Imaging Physics* (4th ed.). Wiley-Liss.

Huda, W. (2008). *Review of Radiologic Physics* (3rd ed.). Lippincott Williams & Wilkins.

Kremkau, F. W. (2015). Diagnostic Ultrasound: Principles and Instruments (8th ed.). Elsevier.

McQuillen Martensen, R. (2014). *Radiographic Image Analysis* (4th ed.). Elsevier.

Mettler Jr, F. A., & Guiberteau, M. J. (2011). *Essentials of Nuclear Medicine Imaging* (6th ed.). Elsevier.

Mitchell, C., & Haroun, L. (2018). Introduction to the Role of Medical Imaging in Diagnosis and Treatment. Oxford University Press.

Prokop, M., Galanski, M., & Schaefer-Prokop, C. (2003). *Spiral and Multislice Computed Tomography of the Body*. Thieme.

Ramachandran, R., & Swamiathan, V. (2016). Diagnostic Radiology: Recent Advances and Applied Physics in Imaging. Jaypee Brothers Medical Publishers.

Samei, E., & Flynn, M. J. (2013). Handbook of Medical Imaging: Volume 1. Physics and Psychophysics. SPIE Press.

Suetens, P. (2009). *Fundamentals of Medical Imaging* (2nd ed.). Cambridge University Press.

Thrall, J. H., & Ziessman, H. A. (2017). *Nuclear Medicine: The Requisites* (4th ed.). Elsevier.

These references are examples of major resources used by radiology professionals. For detailed information on specific subjects, it is recommended to consult these books or other specialist publications in the field of radiology. It is also advisable to consult the latest editions and specialist journals on a regular basis to keep up to date with advances in the field.

Bonnefoy, O., & Favelle, O. (2016). Handbook of radiology for students. Elsevier Masson.

Burgener, F., Kormano, M., & Pudas, T. (2014). *Atlas de poche de Radiologie clinique.* Paris: Flammarion.

Chabrot, P., & Boyer, L. (2018). Cross-sectional imaging of the heart and vessels: Proceedings of the 5th SFC and SFR meetings: Paris, 14-15 March 2013. Springer.

Darai, E., Bazot, M., & Thomassin-Naggara, I. (2015). *Imagerie de la femme.* Paris: Lavoisier.

Delmas, V., & Delmas, A. (2016). Medical anatomy: Fundamental aspects and clinical applications. Paris: Maloine.

Grenier, P., Lacombe, P., & Manelfe, C. (2017). *Imagerie en urgence.* Elsevier Masson.

Hangard, C., & L'Her, P. (2015). *Urgences radiologiques.* Paris: Elsevier.

Menu, Y., & Cadranel, J. (2019). *Digestive imaging.* Paris: Lavoisier.

Perlemuter, L., & Lewin, M. (2018). *Guide clinique d'odontologie.* Paris: Elsevier Masson.

Taourel, P., & Dauzat, M. (2014). *Imagerie du thorax.* Paris: Lavoisier.

Tardivon, A., & Athanasiou, A. (2016). *Breast imaging.* Paris: Lavoisier.

Varoquaux, A., & Barral, M. (2015). *Atlas of genitourinary imaging.* Springer.

Vialle, R., & Dimeglio, A. (2017). *Radiology in orthopaedics.* Elsevier Masson.

The books listed are major French-language references for radiology professionals. For an in-depth understanding of certain subjects, it is recommended that you consult these books or other specialist French-language publications in the field of radiology. To keep up to date with advances and discoveries, it is also advisable to follow recent publications and specialist French-language journals in radiology.

Information on trade associations and conferences

The world of radiology is dense, with numerous professional associations playing a crucial role in the training, certification and professional networking of radiology nurses. These associations also organise conferences to discuss technical, clinical and research advances.

- Professional associations :
  - **Société Française de Radiologie (SFR):** This is one of the largest associations dedicated to radiology in France. It offers a wide range of seminars, training courses and conferences throughout the year.
  - **Association des Manipulateurs en Électroradiologie Médicale (A.F.P.P.M.):** This association is mainly aimed at radiology technologists, but remains a valuable source of information and training for all professionals in the field.
  - **Société Française de Radioprotection (SFRP) (French Radiation Protection Society):** This society focuses on the aspects of radiation protection that are essential for any professional working with radiation.
- Major conferences:
  - **Journées Francophones de Radiologie (JFR):** Organised each year by the SFR, these days bring together professionals from all over the French-speaking world to discuss advances in imaging techniques, diagnostics, etc.
  - **A.F.P.P.M. Congress:** An annual meeting for all medical electroradiology manipulators, offering

workshops, presentations and networking opportunities.

SFRP seminars: Seminars covering all aspects of radiation protection, with presentations by recognised specialists in the field.

Publications and reviews :

La Revue de l'Imagerie Médicale: Published by the SFR, this journal covers all aspects of radiology, with research articles, reviews and case studies.

Radioprotection: This is the official journal of the SFRP. It publishes articles on all aspects of radiation protection, from fundamental research to clinical practice.

Other resources :

Many hospitals, universities and other institutions offer continuing education, webinars and other educational opportunities for radiology professionals.

Online platforms such as Radiopaedia and Medscape can also provide educational resources and updates on the latest developments.

It is strongly recommended that professionals, particularly radiology nurses, join these associations, attend conferences and regularly consult publications to keep up to date in their field.